Aerobics and Fit
Association of America

Exercise
Standards and Guidelines

A Reference Manual for Fitness Professionals

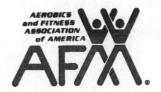

Copyright © 1986, 1989, 1991, 1993, 1995, 1997 by Aerobics and Fitness Association of America,
15250 Ventura Blvd., Suite 200, Sherman Oaks, CA 91403, U.S.A.

ISBN 0-9638168-3-7

Printed in the United States of America

10 9 8 7 6 5 4

Contents

Part I

Basic Exercise Standards and Guidelines

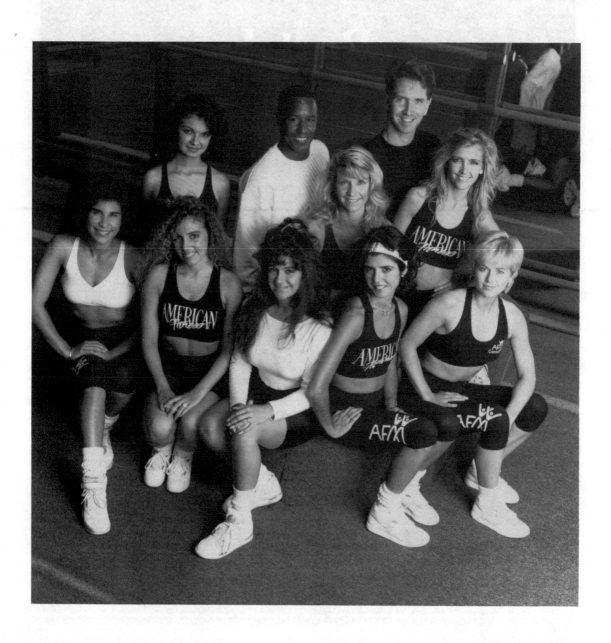

BASIC EXERCISE STANDARDS AND GUIDELINES

of the

Aerobics and Fitness Association of America

These Standards represent an ongoing process of research, critique and consensus by a multidisciplinary team of aerobic fitness industry leaders. Introduced in 1983, the Aerobics and Fitness Association of America's (AFAA's) "Basic Exercise Standards and Guidelines" were the first nationally developed tools used by instructors. This revised 1995 edition reflects a higher level of sophistication and accuracy achieved by applying the most up-to-date research findings to the practice of aerobics.

I. Basic Principles, Definitions and Recommendations

All Standards and Guidelines outlined as follows apply to average adults without known physiological or biological conditions that would in any way restrict their exercise activities.

A. Components of Physical Fitness

A complete physical fitness program should seek to improve and then maintain:

1. Cardiovascular efficiency and endurance

2. Muscular strength and endurance

3. Flexibility

4. Optimal body composition

B. Principles of Training

1. Training Effect

    A **training effect** refers to the physiological changes that occur in the body as a result of exercise. Training should be: (a) consistent, (b) progressive and (c) specific. A training effect will occur if the exercise is sufficient in all of the following areas:

    a. Frequency: number of exercise days per week

    b. Intensity: degrees of physiological stress

    c. Duration: length of time

2. Overload Principle

Training occurs when the body is regularly stimulated beyond its normal workload by progressively increasing **frequency, intensity** and/or **duration** of exercise. The body responds by increasing its capacity to perform work, allowing it to adapt to increasing physiological demands. This principle applies to all types of physical conditioning. This does not mean that you must go for the burn to create a training effect. A **training effect** will occur when muscles are worked slightly beyond their point of fatigue on a regular basis, with periodic increases in **frequency, intensity** and/or **duration** as a result of adaptation to the workload.

3. Specificity of Training

Specificity refers to training specifically for an activity or isolating the specific muscle groups and/or movement pattern that one would like to improve. For example, a marathon runner will train for an event by running distance, not wind sprints, because a marathon is an endurance event. To strengthen a muscle group such as the biceps, choose exercises that isolate the biceps muscles with the least amount of assistance from other muscle groups.

4. Mode of Exercise

Mode of exercise refers to the type of activity that an individual is participating in. Modes of exercise that maintain a consistent intensity level may be more beneficial in improving cardiovascular fitness compared to exercise modes of variable intensities, provided that frequency and duration are also considered.

C. Frequency of Aerobic Training

1. Improving Fitness

Improving fitness is achieved by participating in a minimum of 4-5 aerobic workouts per week. Individuals beginning an exercise program should begin with 3 workouts per week as indicated by qualified exercise prescription. Additional workouts should be added only after an individual has become accustomed to the present level of exercise.

2. Maintaining Fitness

Maintaining fitness is accomplished by a minimum of 3 workouts evenly spaced throughout the week. Detraining occurs within 2 1/2 weeks or less following cessation of exercise, depending upon training level and/or fitness level at the time of exercise cessation.

3. Overtraining

The body needs time to rest, recover and rebuild from the stress of vigorous exercise. Instructors and students should be aware of the following symptoms of overtraining:

a. Fatigue

b. Anemia

4

c. Amenorrhea

d. Stress related injuries

- stress fractures
- tendinitis
- bursitis
- shin splints or other persistent lower leg pain
- chronic knee pain

e. Atypical changes in resting and recovery rates

f. Other symptoms related to weight training

- decrease in strength and lifting performance
- constant soreness leading to pain
- muscle tears

4. Teaching Fitness

As an instructor, be aware of the symptoms of overtraining as outlined above. Individual differences in the number of classes per week that an instructor can teach without risk of overtraining depend on the following variables:

a. Level of fitness

b. Length of time (experience) instructing any one particular type of fitness class

c. Type of class one is teaching

d. Degree of active demonstration

e. Other fitness activities outside of teaching

Twelve classes per week, including no more than two high-impact classes per day, should be the maximum for the experienced instructor.

D. Muscle Balancing

1. Principle

For every primary muscle worked (agonist), the opposing muscle group (antagonist) should also be worked (example: biceps/triceps). By exercising opposing muscle groups, one lessens the possibility of muscular imbalance, thus reducing the potential for injury. Repeating the same exercise month after month works the muscles only through that range of motion, stressing the joint and its attachments in the same areas over and over. A variety of exercises that strengthen both the agonist and antagonist muscle groups will balance and improve joint stability.

2. Muscle Balancing and Posture

Many acquired postural problems (Low Back Syndrome being the most common) may be due to muscular imbalances. These imbalances are manifested by:

   a. Increased lumbar curve

   b. Shortened and contracted iliopsoas

   c. Shortened and contracted hamstrings

   d. Weak abdominals

   e. Hyperextended knees

   f. Rounded upper back and forward shoulders

   g. Supinated or pronated feet

3. Application

Muscular imbalance causes the stronger muscle groups to compensate for the work of the weaker muscles. For example, during a push-up, if the triceps are not equally as strong as the pectoralis muscles in performing the exercise, the pectoralis muscles will take over to perform the majority of the work. Sometimes the agonist muscle can become so much stronger than the antagonist muscle that injury can occur when both the applied stresses to and the support of the skeletal system are unequally distributed among the muscles. For example, in runners, the quadriceps can overpower the strength of the hamstrings causing the hamstrings to become injured due to poor strength ratio between the quadriceps and hamstring muscles.

When muscle imbalances in flexibility and/or strength occur, particularly between anterior and posterior muscles, there is difficulty in maintaining a stabilized torso. To achieve a balanced posture and avoid the risk of Low Back Syndrome:

   a. Strengthen abdominal and quadriceps muscles.

   b. Increase flexibility of back and hamstrings.

   c. Lengthen and release iliopsoas with posterior pelvic tilts and proper stretches for these muscles.

   d. Stand and exercise, maintaining proper body alignment (see following section E—Body Alignment).

   e. Perform exercises regularly for optimum strengthening/lengthening training effect.

   f. Include exercises that concentrate on balance, posture and kinesthetic awareness.

   g. Incorporate muscle isolation techniques to promote torso and pelvic stabilization.

   h. Avoid hyperextension of the knee while standing as this tilts the top of the pelvis forward (anterior), causing the lower back to arch.

   i. Avoid arching or back bends as these activities compress the lumbar spine, possibly resulting in pain and/or damage to the vertebral discs.

   j. Incorporate exercises which functionally strengthen back muscles into a weekly exercise program.

E. Body Alignment

When performing any exercise, be conscious of body alignment and posture. Stand tall, yet keep posture relaxed, not tense. Imagine a "midline" running from the top of the head down through the middle of the body. Keep body weight balanced and evenly distributed in relation to this imaginary "midline." Abdominal muscles should be contracted with rib cage lifted so pelvis is in a neutral alignment with the tailbone pointing down. Shoulders are back and relaxed. Do not hyperextend (lock) knee or elbow joints. Hyperextension places excess stress on ligaments and tendons that attach at each joint, increasing potential for injury as well as decreasing the effectiveness of stretching or strengthening activities.

F. Speed, Isolation and Resistance

Exercises should be performed at a slow to moderate speed that will allow full range of motion and concentrated work for the isolated muscles which are the focus of the exercise. Isolation of a muscle requires that an exercise be specific to the joint action (e.g., flexion, extension, abduction) that will cause a muscle to contract in order to perform work. In order to isolate a muscle group, it is important not to work a muscle beyond the point of fatigue so the other muscle groups compensate and take over to continue work.

An exercise performed too quickly often relies on momentum, making controlled movement impossible, and possibly leading to joint and muscle injury. Strengthening a muscle requires working the muscle against resistance in a controlled, deliberate manner. Resistance is supplied in one of two ways.

1. Through the use of hand-held weights (see AFAA's "Standards and Guidelines for Weighted Workouts"), surgical tubing, elastic bands or other resistive equipment.

2. By concentrating the tension of muscular contraction in the most advantageous position against gravity.

6. Full Range of Motion

1. Normal Range of Motion

    The full degree of movement that a lever is capable of is restricted by the joint and surrounding tissues. Full range of motion is desirable because (a) muscle strength will increase when taken through the entire range of motion of an exercise and (b) it maintains adequate joint mobility.

2. Application

    The working muscle(s) should extend through the full range of motion dictated by the flexibility of the muscles and joint(s) involved. Proper form and body alignment should be maintained and hyperextension should be avoided. To work the muscles efficiently, move through the full range of motion required to complete each exercise.

II. Class Format

A. Sequence

This is a guideline for class design and format that is physiologically sound and effective, and can be appropriately adapted to fit most club policies or personal preference. Only in certain exercise categories, such as warm-up or cool-down, are the specific exercise types important. The following is a recommended sequence used by AFAA for a one-hour class:

1. Pre-class Instruction

2. Warm-up: a balanced combination of rhythmic limbering exercises and static stretching

3. Exercises from the following groups, performed in a standing position, in order of preference:

    a. Aerobics and post-aerobic cool-down

    b. Upper body strengthening

    c. Standing lower body strengthening

4. Descending to the floor for the remainder of the class, exercises from the following groups may be performed in order of preference:

    a. Legs

    b. Buttocks

    c. Hips

    d. Abdominals

    e. Lower back

5. Cool-down: Static Stretching

B. Purpose of Consistent Sequencing

If the above sequence is followed in the order listed, it will be effective because it helps keep the flow of the class smooth. Getting up and down off the floor repeatedly creates "exercise gaps" and can cause rise and fall of heart rate within the aerobic segment, which could have some contraindicated effects. Strive for smooth transitions between exercise activities. Repeatedly stopping class is not only choppy and inconsistent but also a sure way to lose the interest of the class. Keeping the class moving will maintain students' energy and interest levels. The following recommendations should be adhered to regardless of class format:

1. Always begin class with a warm-up.

2. During the aerobic portion, movement should be continuous without abrupt stopping and starting, or peak high and low activity.

3. Always follow aerobics with a sufficient cool-down, including hamstring and calf stretches.

4. Upon completion of strengthening exercises within specific muscle groups, always stretch those muscles before proceeding to the next group.

5. Always end class with static stretching.

C. Class Level

Unless class level is specific, e.g., beginner or advanced, it is best to teach at an intermediate level and explain to the class how to adjust or modify the individual exercises to their particular level of fitness and experience. In other words, try to give both a beginner and advanced version of your exercises while performing at an intermediate level. Skill level, intensity and duration capabilities of individuals must be considered.

III. Instructional Methods, Concerns and Responsibilities

A. Monitoring—Purpose

1. Maximizing Exercise Effectiveness

2. Injury Prevention

   a. Monitoring your students for alignment or performance errors is important in preventing musculoskeletal injury.

   b. Know the following Exercise Danger Signs. Should you observe any one of these or should a class participant complain of any of these, he/she should stop vigorous exercise immediately. If necessary, refer to on-site emergency procedures.

   - unusual fatigue
   - nausea
   - dizziness
   - tightness or pain in the chest
   - lightheadedness
   - loss of muscle control
   - severe breathlessness
   - allergic reactions, e.g., rash or hives
   - blurring of vision

   An individual with any of these symptoms should contact his/her physician and obtain immediate medical advice. It is important that instructors always maintain current CPR certification.

B. Cueing

It is essential that vocal commands are used while instructing. A routine seems to flow more smoothly when the class is verbally cued as to what the next exercise will be.

Anticipatory cues are key words and small phrases which describe an exercise or a sequence which will be performed next. It is also important when teaching exercise that you strongly concentrate on body alignment. An exercise that is done incorrectly may not only be unsafe, but may lack any real benefit. It is essential that you as an instructor give **body alignment cues** for every exercise and make the necessary verbal corrections during class. Hand and directional signals are equally important so you can **visually cue** your class along with verbal cues for clarity.

C. Legal Responsibilities

1. Instructors should complete training and certification programs that test both theoretical knowledge and performance skills and should practice according to the nationally accepted standard.

2. Instructors should carry a personal liability insurance policy.

3. It may be advisable for instructors and club owners to consult an attorney to prepare a participant disclaimer and release that are in accordance with the state and local laws.

4. It may be advisable for fitness facilities and independent fitness contractors to seek program review by qualified fitness and medical professionals.

IV. Pre-Class Procedures

A. Medical Clearance

Before class, determine if there are any new class members and the level of their experience. Ask participants to let you know if they have a medical condition so you can assist them in modifying their workout.

According to the American College of Sports Medicine (ACSM), men under the age of 40 and women under the age of 50 with one risk factor or less and apparently healthy, can participate in moderate exercise without medical clearance.

Medical clearance from a physician prior to exercise participation is recommended for:

- men above the age of 40 and women above the age of 50, regardless of current physical health or risk factors

- anyone with a preexisting medical condition

- anyone with 2 or more risk factors

- anyone with known cardiovascular or other related metabolic disease

- anyone with symptoms suggestive of possible cardiopulmonary or metabolic disease, e.g., chest pain, known heart murmur

Diagnostic exercise testing may be recommended in any of the above instances.

In most cases, if an individual exhibits one or less risk factor, medical clearance is not needed. However, each participant's health and risk factors should be considered individually when determining the need for a medical exam and/or diagnostic exercise testing. At any age, exercise test results provide valuable information, useful in developing a safe and effective exercise prescription. AFAA recommends that an instructor use common sense in relation to risk factors and medical clearance recommendations, as some risk factors may be more significant than others. For example, an individual with high blood pressure or diabetes may be more at risk beginning exercise without clearance than someone who is overweight. It is advisable that all individuals sign a health release and waiver form, indicating their current physical condition as well as medical history prior to exercising.

1. Risk Factors

   Some medical limitations and lifestyle habits require modified programs and specific recommendations. An individual who demonstrates or acknowledges two or more of the following should be advised to have a medical exam and diagnostic exercise test prior to beginning an exercise program:

   - diagnosed high blood pressure*
   - high cholesterol*
   - cigarette smoking*
   - diabetes mellitus*
   - family history of coronary disease or other atherosclerotic disease in parents or siblings prior to the age of 55*
   - sedentary lifestyle (physical inactivity)*
   - obese or overweight
   - high triglycerides and/or abnormal HDL ratio
   - poor eating habits
   - high resting heart rate

   When two or more risk factors are present, extra precautions must be taken prior to exercising as some activities may need to be modified.

2. Effects of Drugs and/or Medications

   Certain prescription as well as non-prescription medications, such as antihistamines and antibiotics, will elicit side effects during exercise similar to the Exercise Danger Signs listed in section III.A,2b of this chapter. Some medications can alter heart rates. For example, beta blockers suppress heart rate activity. It is not recommended that individuals engage in vigorous activity when taking drugs or medication if not under medical supervision. Individuals desiring to continue their exercise regimen should be advised to consult their physician regarding possible side effects.

---

* indicates a major coronary risk factor (according to the ACSM)

B. Introductions

Introduce yourself and announce the level of the class.

C. Attire

If some class members are without shoes, AFAA strongly recommends they obtain and use shoes designed for aerobic exercise as a means of reducing the risk of injury to feet, knees and shins. This should be explained to the class.

D. Level of Participation

Explain that the class is non-competitive and each participant should work at his/her own level. Make sure the class is aware of the Exercise Danger Signs outlined in section III.A,2b of this chapter. In case of any acute pain experienced while exercising, the activity should be discontinued and the instructor should be notified immediately. If any stress or discomfort is experienced by a participant during class, urge him/her to discuss this with you, the instructor, following class.

E. Breathing

Breathing should follow a consistent rhythmic pattern throughout the class. The level of activity will reflexively dictate rate and depth of ventilation. Do not restrict inhalation to the nose. Inhale and exhale through the nose and mouth in a relaxed fashion. Holding your breath while exercising may induce the Valsalva maneuver. The Valsalva maneuver occurs upon the closing of the glottis which creates an unequal pressure in the chest cavity leading to a rise in blood pressure. By the same token, hyperventilating or breathing too hard while exercising can irritate the nasal passage as well as cause lightheadedness.

F. Orientation to Aerobics

Define aerobics for new members (see section VI.A of this chapter). Explain before class how they can calculate their own estimated training heart rate range for aerobic work and how and where to take a pulse count (see section VI.I of this chapter). Explain perceived exertion and how to correlate how one feels with actual exercise intensity.

V. Warm-Up

A. Purpose

Prepares the body for vigorous exercise and may reduce the risk of injury.

B. Time

Class should begin with 8-12 minutes of a balanced combination of static stretches and smoothly performed rhythmic, limbering exercises.

C. Stretching

Correctly performed mild stretching will increase the capacity for full range of movement. This allows one to perform exercises more efficiently with less risk of injury to joint attachments and connective tissue.

1. Muscle Length

    a. Resting length—length of a muscle at rest.

    b. Maximum length—the degree to which a muscle length can be stretched at any particular time.

    c. Increasing length—repeated stretching of a muscle over a period of time will gradually increase the resting length of the muscle fibers.

2. Static Stretch

    Stretches should always be static and non-ballistic. **Static stretches** are sustained in a supportive position which allows the muscle being stretched to relax and elongate. **Ballistic movement** is forcefully executed, causing muscle contraction. Ballistic movement, such as vigorous bouncing during a stretch, invokes the stretch reflex. Stretching is most effective if it is done slowly and gently without bouncing or pulsing.

    Pulsing, though it is a small controlled movement, still elicits muscle contraction and the stretch reflex. Therefore, pulsing is an inappropriate activity to be included during the warm-up.

3. Stretch Reflex

    The stretch reflex is a neurological response, activated as the body's automatic protective mechanism against sudden changes in muscle length, severe injury and abuse. Whenever a muscle is stretched quickly and with force, or beyond the limits of the body's flexibility, an involuntary reflex is initiated by proprioceptors located in the tendon of the muscle being stretched, causing the affected muscle to contract to protect itself and prevent injury and over-stretching.

4. Position

    Always assume a position with the body correctly aligned and supported so the stretch will occur along the muscle's longitudinal line. For example, during a calf stretch, do not rotate the hips and turn the back foot out. Both feet should face the same direction so hips are square to the front leg and a calf stretch can be performed.

5. How to Stretch

    Begin slowly in an easy stretch, not taking the muscle to its maximum length. Stretch to the point of mild tension and hold the position. As the muscle relaxes, increase the stretch slightly until point of tension is reached again. If tension is painful, ease off slightly. Breathing should be slow, rhythmic and controlled. The length of time that a stretch is held will vary according to whether or not one is stretching at the beginning of class when the muscles are not thoroughly prepared, or at the end of class when the muscles are warm. For warm-up, hold each stretch approximately 8-10 seconds. Avoid stretching muscles that are cold prior to performing certain preliminary rhythmic limbering exercises.

D. Sequence

In order to maintain a smooth flow to your warm-up, follow an order that will include all major muscle groups. Warming up from either head to toes, or vice versa, is an easy way to avoid omitting any muscle groups.

E. Muscle Groups

AFAA recommends all of the following muscle groups be warmed up at the beginning of class, depending on class type and format:

1. Head and neck (sternocleidomastoid, levator scapula, trapezius-occipital portion)

2. Upper back, middle back, rib cage, shoulders (trapezius, rhomboids, latissimus dorsi, teres major, serratus anterior, anterior, medial and posterior deltoid, and rotator cuff muscles)

3. Chest and arms (pectoralis major and minor, biceps brachii, triceps brachii, brachioradialis, brachialis)

4. Front of torso and lower back (rectus abdominis, external and internal obliques, erector spinae)

5. Front and back of thighs (quadriceps group and sartorius, hamstring group)

6. Buttocks (gluteus maximus)

7. Outer thigh and upper hip (tensor fascia latae, gluteus medius and minimus)

8. Inner thigh (adductors longus, brevis and magnus; pectineus and gracilis)

9. Calf and front of shin (gastrocnemius, soleus, tibialis anterior)

10. Feet and ankles (flexors and extensors)

F. Rhythmic Limbering Exercises

Rhythmic limbering exercises are multi-joint exercises that incorporate large muscle groups and are performed at a smooth and moderate pace. They help prepare your body for more vigorous exercise by increasing the range of motion of the joint and its attachments, raising muscle and body temperature, increasing circulation to the tissues surrounding the joints, and maximizing neuromuscular function. Rhythmic limbering exercises can serve as a rehearsal of similar moves that may be performed later at a higher exercise intensity.

G. Special Do's and Don'ts

1. **Do** rhythmically warm-up and static stretch the lower back before attempting lateral spinal flexion or spinal rotation, in which one arm, straight or bent, would diagonally (by lifting or reaching) cross the sagittal plane or body's midline.

2. **Don't** do traditional toe touches to stretch the hamstrings as these place a strain on the lower back muscles and ligaments.

3. **Don't** do full deep knee bends (grand pliés) as these strain the cruciate ligaments in the knees. **Do** keep hips above knee level.

4. **Don't** do rapid head rolls or hyperextend the cervical spine as these movements strain the neck muscles and place tension on the vertebrae and discs in the cervical region.

H. Special Considerations

1. Spinal Flexion—Forward

   Although the spine was meant to flex forward, hanging with the torso in an unsupported position with gravity pulling downward on the back can place stress on the vertebrae, discs and connective tissue (e.g., ligaments) in the lumbar region as well as increase potential for overstretching lower back muscles and ligaments of the spine. Ligaments have little elasticity. Once overstretched, they remain elongated, decreasing the stability and support in the lumbar region.

   Follow these guidelines if you choose to perform exercises in the spinal forward flexed position:

   a. When stretching or performing rhythmic limbering exercises, all movements should be performed in a controlled manner.

   b. Do not maintain any forward flexed position for an extended period of time as overstretching of the ligaments in the lower back may occur.

   c. Always support the torso by flexing from the hip joint, placing hands on the upper leg above the knee joint, lower leg or directly on the floor, depending upon individual flexibility level. Avoid arching backward.

   d. Contract abdominals to protect the lower back. By keeping the torso stabilized with a neutral spine, the internal organs are supported by the abdominal muscles to maintain a correct posture.

   e. Keep hips above knee level when flexing at both hip and knee joints. Allowing the hips to drop below the knees places stress on the ligaments of the knee as well as the back.

   f. Always roll up from a bent over position, with knees relaxed.

   g. When stretching hamstrings from a standing or seated position, lead with the chest and bend from the hips. Do not bend from the waist or back, arch the back or drop the head. Head should always be in alignment with spine.

2. Spinal Flexion—Lateral

Unsupported stretching to the side for a long period of time can be just as stressful as anterior spinal flexion if performed incorrectly. These positions can be potentially dangerous and can cause ligament damage. Individuals who can stretch sideways to a horizontal position are usually relying on ligaments that have been overstretched in past activities by forcing or bouncing to increase flexibility.

Follow these guidelines when performing any type of lateral stretch:

a. Support the torso with one hand on torso or thigh with hips squared.

b. Never lean so far over to the side that you are "hanging" and have to throw one hip out of alignment to support the back.

c. Do not perform lateral flexion with both hands extended over head.

VI. Aerobics

A. Definition and Purpose

Aerobic exercise can be defined as a variety of activities which create an increased demand for oxygen over an extended period of time. Aerobic exercises train the cardiovascular and respiratory systems to exchange and deliver oxygen quickly and efficiently to every part of the body being exercised. As the heart muscle becomes stronger and more efficient, a larger volume of blood is able to be pumped with each stroke and with fewer strokes, thus facilitating the rapid transport of oxygen to all parts of the body with less stress on the heart. An aerobically fit cardiovascular system will allow an individual to work longer, at a more vigorous pace, with a quicker recovery.

B. Time

A minimum of 20-30 minutes of continuous activity is recommended.

C. Sequence

The aerobic portion should resemble a normal bell curve. Start slowly and gradually increase the intensity and range of motion of your aerobic movements. Avoid lateral high-impact moves such as pendulum leg swings, jumping jacks or high-impact grapevines during the first three minutes to allow your ankles and feet to become sufficiently warmed up. Peak movements, which involve a larger range of motion using both arms and legs, require a greater amount of oxygen to be delivered to the muscles and should be interspersed with lower-intensity aerobic patterns to maintain a steady state. These peak movements should not be included during the first three minutes.

D. Position

Correct posture (see section I.E of this chapter), with the abdominals contracted and rib cage lifted, should be maintained throughout the aerobic portion. For all exercises performed, heels should contact the floor with each step. When jogging, follow these guidelines:

1. **Don't** jog on your toes, as this shortens the calf muscles and Achilles tendon.

2. **Don't** lean forward, as this can contribute to shin splints and knee stress.

3. **Do** keep body weight balanced over entire foot and not backward on heels.

4. **Don't** kick heel up to touch buttocks, as this arches the lower back. Keep knees aligned under or in front of hips.

E. **Types of Movements**

Try to vary your movements in order to maintain interest level and effectively involve as many muscles as possible. Combination moves requiring coordination of both arms and legs should be entered into slowly, starting with either the arms or the legs and then adding the other. Build upon your moves instead of trying to teach a complicated combination all at once. Choose moves that are appropriate for the fitness level of the class. Avoid extended periods of jumping or high leg kicks. Do not jump on the same leg more than 8 times in succession because of risk of injury caused by repeated impact. Avoid elevating the arms overhead for an extended period of time as this activates the pressor response (the heart rate and blood pressure are elevated disproportionately to the oxygen cost of the activity).

F. **Breathing**

Steady, rhythmic breathing through both the nose and mouth should be maintained. Holding one's breath should be avoided.

G. **Surface**

Aerobics should ideally be performed on a suspended wood floor, which provides a cushion of air between wood and concrete, or on high density mat-type aerobic flooring. If jogging on concrete is unavoidable, mats should be used or low-impact movements should be utilized.

H. **Music Speed**

AFAA recommends music speed during the aerobic portion range from 130-155 beats per minute (bpm), depending upon fitness level and type of activity (e.g., high-impact, low-impact, a combination of high- and low-impact, and low-impact with weights). When selecting music speed, lever length (e.g., arms, legs and torso) needs to be considered so individuals can complete a full range of motion for an exercise at that given speed.

I. **Heart Rate**

Monitoring heart rate serves as a guideline recommendation, indicating the level of exertion (intensity) for each participant.

1. Where to Take Pulse

    a. **Radial artery**: Place the fingers on the inner wrist, just below the wrist bon
        straight down from the base of thumb. This location is preferred to the caroti
        pulse due to the possible depressant effect on the heart rate during palpation a
        the carotid site.

    b. **Carotid artery**: Place index and middle fingers on outside corner of eye and slid
        them straight down to the neck. Do not press hard or place thumb on opposite
        side of neck at the same time, as the blood flow could be impeded and accurate
        heart rate measurements would not be possible.

2. How to Determine Your Heart Rate

    a. **Count**—Count your pulse for 10 seconds, beginning with "1."

    b. **Multiply**—Multiply this number by 6, and you will know what your estimated
        heart rate is for 1 minute at that particular time.

3. Resting Heart Rate

    a. **Averages**—Average for women is 78-84 bpm. Average for men is 72-78 bpm. A
        person in good aerobic condition generally has a lower resting heart rate.

    b. **How to determine your resting heart rate**—Take pulse for three consecutive
        mornings while still lying down, but after heart rate has settled down if awakened
        by an alarm. Add these three numbers together and then divide the answer by
        3. This number is your resting heart rate.

4. Maximum Heart Rate

    Maximum heart rate (MHR) is the theoretical maximum number at which your heart
    can beat at your age, based on the maximum heart rate of a baby at birth. The
    mathematical constant, 220 minus your age, equals your **estimated** maximum heart
    rate. **Do not exercise at this level!**

5. Training Heart Rate Range

    a. **Purpose**—Provides an easily identifiable gauge of an individual's level of aerobic
        work and whether or not the intensity of aerobic activities should be increased
        or decreased.

    b. **To determine your training heart rate range** (THRR), subtract your age from
        220 and multiply this number by .55 and .85. This is your training heart rate
        range or zone that you should "target" during aerobic exercise. Individuals with
        special needs (e.g., pregnant women or anyone with a history of cardiorespiratory
        problems) should consult a physician regarding the recommended training heart
        rate range. When beginning an aerobics program, it is recommended that all
        individuals train at the lower end of their range for the first 8 to 10 weeks.

6. Application

    The pulse should be quickly located after vigorous exercise. Keep feet moving by
    stepping in place or walking, and take a 10-second count. Multiply by 6. This number
    should be in your individualized training range. If it is higher or lower than the

recommended limits of your range, you will need to adjust the intensity of your exercise accordingly by being more or less vigorous.

7. Monitoring Heart Rate During Exercise

In the most ideal of situations, AFAA recommends taking heart rate at 3 different times: (1) 5 minutes after the beginning of active aerobic work to determine if the participant is exercising within his/her training heart rate range; (2) at the completion of the most intense aerobic work to see if he/she has maintained aerobic training level; and (3) at the completion of post-aerobic cool-down to determine if he/she has sufficiently recovered from aerobic work. However, as taking heart rates at these times is not always feasible, heart rate should be checked at the completion of the most intense aerobic work rather than not at all.

8. Recovery Heart Rate

A recovery heart rate can indicate an individual's fitness level by the speed at which heart rate returns to a pre-exercise level. It is also an indicator of whether the cool-down period was sufficient, and if exercise intensity was appropriate. After 5 minutes, the heart rate should be 60% or less of the estimated maximum heart rate (220 minus age, multiplied by .6).

VII. Post-Aerobic Cool-Down

A. Purpose

A post-aerobic cool-down provides a transitional period between vigorous aerobic work and muscular strengthening exercises or stretches. Without a gradual cool-down period, the blood can pool in the extremities immediately after an aerobic workout and does not return to the heart quickly or efficiently if movement stops suddenly. Moderate to slow rhythmic movements for the upper and lower body will enable the muscles of the extremities to pump the blood back to the heart and brain. Stopping motionless after an aerobic workout could result in lightheadedness and/or fainting.

B. Time

Approximately 2-3 minutes of decreased intensity aerobic work such as walking, marching or other rhythmic activities is recommended.

C. Breathing

Breathing should be relaxed with rate and depth dictated by physiological reflexes. Students should learn to be aware of their own oxygen requirements and learn to regulate their breathing accordingly.

D. Stretches

After 2-3 minutes, muscles that have been utilized during the aerobic portion (especially the calves, front of lower leg, quadriceps, hip flexors, hamstrings and the back) should be statically stretched for 10-20 seconds before proceeding with other exercises or rest.

E. Heart Rate

As an added precaution, AFAA recommends that the heart rate be checked again before beginning floorwork. Heart rate should not exceed 60% of estimated maximum heart rate (220 minus age, multiplied by .6) 5 minutes after aerobic work ceases. If heart rate is too high, continue walking slowly until heart rate has lowered sufficiently.

VIII. Upper Body Exercises

A. Purpose

To strengthen and improve muscle endurance of the arms, chest, shoulders and back.

B. Time

Approximately 5-7 minutes is recommended.

C. Isolating Upper Body Exercises

Exercises may be performed with the lower body in a stationary position, with limited lower body movement, or may be incorporated with the aerobics. If performed during the aerobic portion, keep footwork simple so the upper body muscle groups may be the area of concentrated work. Always include exercises that will work the opposing muscle groups for muscle balancing.

D. Method

See section I.F, 1 and 2 (Speed, Isolation and Resistance) of this chapter.

E. Position

In a standing, stationary position maintain correct body alignment. Abdominals should be contracted, rib cage lifted, knees relaxed with pelvis in neutral alignment. The same upper body alignment should be applied when performing arm work during aerobics. Do not use momentum as this can alter both the effectiveness of the exercise as well as body alignment, placing unnecessary strain on the back muscles. Do not hyperextend elbow or shoulder joints, but do move through the fullest range of motion that is possible for maximum muscle involvement. Choose exercises that will work muscle(s) in the most advantageous position against gravity. Use alternate positions to standing (e.g., kneeling, lunging, sitting, supine, prone) for variety as well as torso stabilization.

F. Push-ups

Push-ups, performed with either straight legs or on the knees, can be excellent exercises for strengthening the muscles of the arms and chest. In order to perform push-ups safely, the following guidelines should be noted:

1. To protect the lower back, it is advisable to raise the buttocks slightly when the legs are fully extended, maintaining a neutral pelvic tilt.

2. Hands should be positioned on the floor, even with shoulders or slightly outside shoulder width.

3. Hand placement should be slightly forward of shoulders with fingers pointing straight ahead comfortably, following the natural curve of an individual's arms as they are extended. When hands are rotated inward or outward, it increases the amount of stress to wrist and elbow joints, and changes the muscle groups being exercised.

4. Elbows should not lock or overbend.

5. Head should be held straight in a natural extension of the spine.

6. Body weight should be evenly balanced, regardless of position, by distributing support between arms, upper torso and legs. This will minimize stress to the shoulders, wrist joints and lower back.

7. Both the descent and ascent should be performed as a smooth movement, so that the body's line remains straight without sagging in the middle. Lead with the chest, not the abdominals.

8. When push-ups are performed on the knees, knees should be directly under or behind hips, depending on fitness level.

9. In any position, separate the legs for balance and lower body weight distribution.

G. Torso Stabilization

Mild to moderate lower back strengthening and conditioning will occur when back muscles are involved to directly stabilize the torso as exercises for other muscle groups are performed, e.g., squats, standing hip extensions. It is important to strengthen these muscles because they hold the torso in pelvic neutral alignment. Strengthening back muscles that are not directly involved in holding the torso in a neutral position, but are utilized for all lifting and bending activities, should also be performed as indirect stabilization exercises, e.g., bent over rows, lat pulls, reverse pliés. Strengthening back muscles both directly and indirectly can aid in reducing risk of back injury. Be aware of the following guidelines:

1. When performing exercises that utilize lower back muscles, be conscious of proper form and alignment.

2. Always maintain pelvic neutral alignment and an erect torso when performing any exercises.

3. When bending forward, flex at the hip joint instead of flexing the spine which rounds the back, as this will stress the lower back and pull on back ligaments.

4. Don't hyperextend the spine in an unsupported position when the spine is not stabilized.

5. Individuals who experience back pain or have a history of chronic back pain should be advised by a medical professional as to which exercises are appropriate for them.

    Back strengthening can also be performed in a prone position (see section X of this chapter).

IX. Legs, Hips and Buttocks Exercises

A. Purpose

To strengthen the muscles of the legs, hips and buttocks.

B. Time

Approximately 10-15 minutes is recommended.

C. Hips and Outer Thigh—Side-lying Position

1. Primary Muscles and Joint Action

   Gluteus medius and minimus, tensor fascia latae: hip abduction

2. Alignment and Method

   Body should be in a straight line, either lying fully extended on the floor or raised up on one elbow with supporting arm positioned squarely on the floor under shoulder; rib cage should be lifted so that torso does not collapse. For either position, shoulders and hips should remain square during the execution of any of the exercise variations, with the hips neither leaning to the front nor rolling backward. Use top arm to help stabilize the upper body. Lower leg should be relaxed and both legs aligned so knees can "stack" when both legs are extended in a straight line. Position of the bottom leg is for support only and may change with different exercise variations. When extending the upper leg, extend directly to the side without locking the knee.

   To isolate the outer thigh and hip muscles, resistance should be on the upward lift against gravity and not the downward motion. Lift the leg as high as possible without altering alignment. The knee should face forward during the entire exercise. If the knee points "upward," either basic alignment has altered by leaning backward onto hip or hip rotators are actively involved in the movement.

   a. Special Considerations—"L" Position

      The "L" position requires the upper leg or both legs to be placed in a position at 90 degrees in relationship to the upper torso. For this reason, AFAA does not recommend the use of the "L" position as it strains the gluteus medius tendon and is difficult to maintain if an individual has inflexible hamstrings. Place legs, either bent or straight, at a 45-degree angle to the hips for a more appropriate variation.

3. Common Problems

   * rolling back on hip

   * supporting elbow too close or too far out from shoulder

   * arching of the lower back

   * "slouching" on supporting arm, causing the rib cage to collapse rather than be lifted

- lifting top leg too high, throwing the body out of alignment
- using momentum rather than controlled resistance
- rolling hips too far forward
- twisting upper torso so shoulders are not square
- intermediate position (side-lying, unsupported sagging torso and/or cervical spine; elbow in contact with floor and head resting in hand)

D. Hips and Outer Thigh—All-fours Position

1. Primary Muscles and Joint Action

   Gluteus medius and minimus, tensor fascia latae: hip abduction.

2. Alignment and Method

   On all fours, when working one leg to the side, knees should be separated and aligned under hips with hands under shoulders. Hands and fingers should face forward and elbows should be slightly relaxed, not locked. Hips remain square, pelvis in neutral alignment and weight should be balanced evenly between supporting leg and leg to be lifted. Do not lean to the side to compensate for lack of strength or to achieve greater height. Abdominals should be contracted with pelvis tilted so that the lower back doesn't arch. Head should be held in a natural extension of the spine, not hanging down.

   Raise bent leg directly to the side. Knee remains pointing forward. Lift the leg only as high as possible with the hips square and without leaning over onto the supporting leg. Do not perform straight leg lifts directly to the side. This position stresses the lower back and supporting hip and is difficult to perform while maintaining proper body alignment. All abduction work performed in this position should be slow and controlled without using momentum to gain height. Modifying this position to elbows and knees does not allow enough range of motion against gravity, nor does it effectively work primary muscles involved, particularly for an individual with long levers.

3. Common Problems
   - leaning to one side
   - using momentum to lift leg
   - lifting leg too high and not directly to side
   - dropping head down
   - using torso movement rather than isolating the leg that is being lifted
   - arching lower back (sway back)
   - locking elbows

E. Inner Thigh—Side-lying Position

1. Primary Muscles and Joint Action

   Adductors longus, brevis and magnus; gracilis, pectineus: hip adduction

2. Alignment and Method

   Body should be in a straight line, shoulders and hips are square. The most effective position is to lie all the way down with head resting on forearm, top leg in a supportive position so that foot, ankle and knee are aligned. The position of the top leg can either be all the way down on the floor or with the knee slightly elevated, depending on lever length and ability to maintain a position so that hips aren't rolling forward or backward. This allows inner thigh to be isolated with the bottom leg extended directly to the side in a straight line with the torso.

   Movement of the inner leg is upward against gravity. If using a position where the torso is raised and supported by forearm, maintain this position without collapsing torso as the lower leg is lifted.

3. Common Problems
   - rolling hips back so body weight is on buttocks
   - holding bottom leg either too far forward or too far behind torso; should be extended directly to the side
   - turning toe of bottom leg upward so that the quadriceps are involved or turning the toe downward so that the hamstrings are involved
   - top leg position places too much stress on ankle and knee joints
   - intermediate position (side-lying, unsupported sagging torso and/or cervical spine; elbow in contact with floor and head resting in hand)

F. Inner Thigh—Supine Position

1. Primary Muscles and Joint Action

   Adductors longus, brevis and magnus; gracilis, pectineus: hip adduction.

2. Alignment and Method

   Lie on back with legs vertically raised in air above hips, shoulder width apart. Knees may be bent or only slightly relaxed. If legs are too far apart, it requires the use of the hip flexors to bring the legs close enough together to isolate the inner thigh muscles, which may cause the back to arch off the floor. If legs are straight, don't lock at the knee joint.

   Bring legs together, resisting motion in toward body's midline. Place hands either on inside of thighs for added resistance, or relaxed at sides. It is important to control speed so that the exercise remains resistive without the use of momentum. If an individual places his/her hands under hips to lift pelvis, it is difficult to maintain vertical alignment of the legs over the hips if abdominals are weak. Placing hands under hips forces pelvis into an unnatural position if individual cannot naturally support lifted legs unaided. An individual should be able to maintain correct position required for this exercise with his/her own body strength and flexibility.

3. Common Problems

- arching the lower back off the floor
- using ballistic moves outward, rather than resisting in toward midline of body
- legs dropping too far forward, causing strain on lower back

G. Buttocks—All-fours Position

1. Primary Muscles and Joint Action

   Gluteus maximus: hip extension

2. Alignment and Method

   On all fours, when working one leg extended to the rear, the hips should be square and the back straight, not swayed. Knees should be separated and aligned under hips with hands under shoulders. Abdominals should be contracted. Head is in alignment with the spine and elbows are slightly bent, not hyperextended. This position can be modified to elbows and knees; the same alignment applies. If using elbow and knee position, elbows should be positioned under shoulders.

   Leg lifts should be performed through full range of motion without lifting leg above hip height. Movement should be upward without torso involvement. Avoid jerking or throwing the leg upward as this can stress the lower back. Balance weight between supporting leg and extended leg. In either recommended position, emphasis is on the "upward" movement against gravity, contracting the gluteals with each lift. Avoid exercises that arch and hyperextend the lower back, or use momentum, such as the donkey kick.

3. Common Problems

- arching the lower back
- raising leg higher than hip in either position
- torso movement
- momentum
- head dropped, abdominals not contracted
- hip laterally rotated so toes point outward, involving the hip rotator muscles

H. Buttocks—Prone Position

1. Primary Muscles and Joint Action

   Gluteus maximus: hip extension

2. Alignment and Method

Lying face down on stomach, with both legs extended, hips and chest should remain in contact with floor, pelvis in neutral alignment and abdominals contracted. To maintain this position, the pelvis must be tilted posteriorly in proper neutral alignment so that the lower back is protected. Head is in a comfortable position, either resting on forearms, chin on floor or neck laterally rotated to face sideways. Variations and movements are the same as recommended for the all-fours and elbow-knee positions. The range of motion in the prone position is limited to avoid hyperextending the back and to keep the hips in contact with the floor throughout the entire movement. For isolation of the buttocks, don't do double leg lifts as this stresses the vertebrae, ligaments and muscles in lower back.

3. Common Problems

- arching the lower back
- using the lower back muscles instead of buttocks to perform exercises
- raising leg higher than hips
- hips lifting off floor
- using momentum

I. Buttocks—Supine Position

1. Primary Muscles and Joint Action

   Gluteus maximus: hip extension

2. Alignment and Method

   When lying on back, knees should be bent and feet flat on floor, a comfortable distance from body. Back should not arch but be in contact with floor prior to initial movement. Pelvis should be tilted and abdominals contracted. Arms may be relaxed in any position that is comfortable, e.g., behind head or close to torso.

   The gluteal muscles should be contracted with the upward movement against gravity and released with the downward movement without jerking or bouncing the pelvis up and down. Lift only high enough to lift pelvis off the floor, keeping the mid-back and waist (mid-torso) area in contact with the floor throughout the entire movement.

3. Common Problems

- using back rather than pelvis to lift
- arching lower back off floor
- expanding rib cage
- feet too close to body, stressing knees, or too far from body, arching lower back
- knees not aligned with toes

J. Quadriceps—Standing Position

1. Primary Muscles and Joint Action

   Quadriceps group: rectus femoris, vastus lateralis, vastus intermedius, vastus medialis; sartorius: hip flexion, knee extension

   Hip flexors: psoas major and minor; iliacus: hip flexion

2. Alignment and Method

   In a standing position, use basic guidelines for body alignment (see section I.E of this chapter): knees should be relaxed and aligned in the same direction as the toes, pelvis in neutral alignment, abdominals contracted and rib cage lifted. Shoulders should remain back in a relaxed position.

   a. Squats

   When performing a squat or any squat variation, feet may be placed about shoulder width apart, knees and feet aligned in the same direction. Squat in a controlled manner, lowering torso until thighs are parallel or slightly above parallel to the floor. Hips should never drop below knee level. Overbending or bending too low may cause stress to the ligaments of the knee. During the lowering phase of a squat, the tailbone points to the rear as an extension of the spine, without arching the back. From a squat, straighten legs without hyperextending knees to full extension of the hips to pelvic neutral alignment. Keep lower back in a fixed position without torso movement during entire descent and ascent to reduce overstraining back muscles. Keep heels on floor during entire exercise by balancing body weight evenly over feet. Don't lean forward; keep torso erect.

   b. Pliés

   When performing a plié or "modified squat," feet should be about or slightly more than shoulder distance apart in a comfortable position, with the toes turned outward and aligned with knees. The pelvis is stabilized in neutral alignment with the rib cage lifted and abdominals contracted. Knees should remain slightly flexed. During the lowering phase of a plié, the torso remains in neutral alignment with the tailbone pointing downward. Descend only as low as possible without changing alignment of the pelvis or overshooting the toes with the knees. From a plié, straighten legs without hyperextending knees to full extension of the hips to pelvic neutral alignment. The torso remains erect without leaning forward during both the descent and ascent. Variations with one or both heels lifted may be appropriate as long as proper body alignment can be maintained.

   c. Lunges

   When performing a lunge and any lunge variation, the front knee should never extend beyond toes. This places tremendous strain on the knee joint and its attachments. The lower front leg should be perpendicular to the floor on any lunge variation, whether stationary or moving. Don't step so far forward that the return move places a strain on the back and alters alignment. The depth of the lunge will depend on type of lunge performed. However, don't lunge so deep that the back knee touches the floor or so low that knee pain or strain is felt.

d. Standing Knee Extension/Hip Flexion

When performing standing knee extensions, do not hyperextend or lock the knee. This exercise should be performed in a controlled manner without any rapid jerky motions. Standing exercises can include any variety of knee extension and hip flexion movements in combination or isolation. Doing these exercises in a standing position requires good balance. When performing hip flexion, either with a straight or bent knee, maintain pelvic neutral alignment. Don't lift leg so high that the buttocks "tuck under." This is all hip flexor work with little quadriceps isolation and relies on momentum for leg height. Rotating the hip can isolate different muscles within the quadriceps group. If performing exercises utilizing rotation, the same basic guidelines for standing alignment should be followed.

NOTE: Squats, pliés and lunges are multi-muscle exercises which additionally involve the gluteus maximus and hamstring group.

3. Common Problems

    - using momentum rather than a controlled lift in a standing position

    - hyperextension of the knee joint when performing extensions or straightening knees from a squat position

    - arching the lower back

    - dropping hips below knees during a squat

    - extending knees beyond toes when performing a squat or lunge

    - lifting heels off floor during a squat

    - loss of balance or leaning to one side when performing hip flexion/knee extension variations

K. **Quadriceps—Sitting or Supine Position**

1. Primary Muscles and Joint Action

Quadriceps femoris group: rectus femoris, vastus lateralis, vastus intermedius, vastus medialis; sartorius: hip flexion, knee extension

2. Alignment and Method

Effective quadriceps strengthening can also be accomplished by either sitting in a chair or on the floor, supported on elbows, or lying on the back. For any of these positions, the upper torso should be maintained in a supported position, shoulders back. Keep the non-working leg bent and foot flat on floor for support. If supported on elbows, don't slouch, but keep rib cage lifted, shoulders down and pelvis tilted to press lower back to the floor. Keep abdominals contracted. When lying supine, lower back should remain pressed to the floor for the entirety of the exercise being performed. Sitting upright on the floor and maintaining an erect posture is difficult, and the range of motion of the exercise is limited to decrease the amount of hip flexor work. Use the other alternative positions unless the sitting position can be maintained for a desired number of repetitions and can accomplish muscle fatigue.

Use slow, controlled resistive movement to perform knee extensions or straight leg lifts. To work the entire quadriceps group, both joint actions need to be included as part of a complete strengthening program. As in the standing position, don't lift leg so high that only hip flexors are utilized. Lifting the working leg to approximately knee height of the supporting leg will help to isolate the quadriceps and lessen hip flexor involvement. Going beyond knee height or a 45-degree angle is mostly hip flexor work. Note that rotation of hip will emphasize work of different muscles within the quadriceps group.

3. Common Problems

- using momentum rather than a controlled lift

- hyperextension of the knee joint

- using hip flexors exclusively to lift leg

- slouching in the supported elbow position

- leaning backward in the sitting position

- arching the back in supine position

L. Hamstring—Standing, All-fours and Prone Positions

1. Primary Muscles and Joint Action

Hamstring group: biceps femoris, semitendinosus, semimembranosus: knee flexion, hip extension

2. Alignment and Method

Hamstring strengthening occurs when performing straight leg lifts and bent knee curls behind the body. In order to strengthen the entire hamstring group, both joint actions, particularly knee flexion, need to be included as part of a complete strengthening program. When strengthening hamstrings in a standing position, follow the alignment guidelines outlined for quadriceps in a standing position (see section IX.J of this chapter). Hamstrings will also be strengthened as the opposing muscle group when performing squats. To strengthen hamstrings on all fours or prone, follow the guidelines outlined for buttocks (see section IX.G-H of this chapter). In either of these positions, strengthening will occur by curling the foot toward buttocks or with a controlled straight leg lift in a resistive manner against gravity. To protect the back and isolate hamstring muscles, do not arch the back or lift leg above hip level. Do not rotate the hips, but maintain a "hips square" position.

3. Common Problems

- arching the lower back

- hips not squared; one hip is higher than the other

- no resistance with the curl

- rotating hip outward

- leaning on one leg in all-fours position

- not fully extending legs to complete ascent on a squat

29

X. Lower Back Exercises

A. Purpose

To strengthen the muscles of the lower back.

1. Primary Muscles and Joint Action

Erector spinae: spinal extension

B. Time

Approximately 5-7 minutes is recommended.

C. Alignment and Method—Prone Position

Lying face down on stomach with both legs extended, hips should remain in contact with floor. Maintain a pelvic tilt to keep pelvis in neutral alignment and abdominals contracted. Depending on the variations utilized, arms can either both be extended overhead, one arm extended overhead, extended close to torso or bent with forearms folded to support head. For all variations, the head must remain lowered and the neck should be in good spinal alignment without any hyperextension. To protect the lower back discs and ligaments, the rib cage and chest should be in contact with the floor while performing exercises.

Variations for mild to moderate back strengthening include: (1) lifting one straight leg at a time to hip height, (2) alternating straight leg lifts, (3) lifting one leg and opposite arm or (4) lifting both arms with torso slightly raised while legs remain in contact with the floor. Pelvic neutral alignment should be maintained throughout lifting and lowering phases of exercise so that hips remain in contact with the floor. Avoid lifting both legs at the same time as this variation can rely on momentum if the lower back muscles are weak, and can increase the risk of pressure to the intervertebral discs. Don't place hands under hips as these exercises should be performed only if an individual is strong enough to maintain alignment unaided. A modified cobra position supported on the forearms, held statically for 10-20 seconds can also be utilized. Move slowly with forearms in contact with floor to minimize hyperextension of lower back. Keep head aligned with spine.

D. Common Problems

- using momentum on any variation to gain more height
- lifting head, shoulders and/or upper torso off floor when lifting leg
- double leg lifts
- lifting hips off floor
- hyperextension of the back

XI. Abdominal Exercises

A. Purpose

To strengthen the abdominal muscles and provide support for the internal organs and the back.

1. Primary Muscles and Joint Action

Rectus abdominis: spinal flexion

External and internal obliques: lateral spinal flexion, spinal rotation

Transverse abdominis: abdominal compression

B. Time

Approximately 5-8 minutes is recommended.

C. Alignment and Method—Supine Position

In order to isolate and enervate all four of the abdominal muscles, an abdominal curl which flexes the spine approximately 30-45 degrees will contract these muscles sufficiently to improve strength and tone. Lie on your back on the floor, with knees bent, feet flat on the floor at a comfortable distance away from your body. Tilt pelvis in such a way that the lower back and torso maintain a neutral spinal position so the lower back can be on the floor or as close to the floor as possible without creating an extreme posterior tilt.

1. A curl will bring the head, neck, shoulders and rib cage up and forward in a slow controlled motion without momentum so the scapula clears the floor at the top of the lift. Do not lift with the neck and push the head out of alignment. Head should be fully supported without any neck movement (see arm positions in section XI.D of this chapter). Return to starting position without dropping the head and shoulders on the floor. Maintain a consistent, moderate contraction of the abdominals throughout the exercises performed. Keep the lower back on the floor to stabilize the pelvis and protect the back.

2. Additionally strengthen the external and internal obliques by including exercises that involve rotation with the lower torso stable and motionless. Keeping the lower body stationary when rotating will help to isolate the oblique muscles because resistance will occur against the lower body as a stabilizing force. The hips should not roll from side to side as the torso is lifted. When rotating, lead with the shoulder, not the elbow, so that the twist lifts the upper body in one fluid motion. Elbow motion does not guarantee that torso movement is also taking place.

3. When performing a reverse curl or pelvic thrust, both legs should be elevated with the thighs perpendicular to the hips so that the lift will occur as a result of reverse spinal flexion, not hip flexion. In this position, if these exercises are performed correctly, the hip flexors are deactivated to allow the abdominal muscles to contract,

resulting in a curl of the lower torso toward the chest, or a vertical lift. Maintain no less than a 90-degree angle of the legs to the hips.

Dropping both legs away from the torso below this angle will place stress on the lumbar spine, causing the back to arch. Use these variations only with individuals who are strong enough to maintain alignment and can perform exercises without momentum to initiate the lift.

D. Arm Positions

When supporting the head, do not clasp and interlock fingers behind neck. This position does not offer support if you are pressing forward on neck or if the head hangs down behind neck in a hyperextended position. Place open fingers on the back of head for better support. Arms may also be extended up and/or out in front of the body as long as the head and neck are aligned as an extension of the spine. Other arm variations may include but are not limited to: crossing arms in front of chest; fingers on forehead or top of head with elbows forward; forearms crossed or extended behind head. Avoid always looking up at the ceiling as this position may not correspond to chosen arm position and abdominal exercise. Arm positions should complement the abdominal exercise that is being performed along with modifications for fitness level.

E. Abdominal Work vs. Hip Flexor Work

During a full sit-up, the first 40 degrees of movement rely on the abdominals. However, the remainder of the movement toward a full sitting position depends on the hip flexors (iliopsoas muscles). When lying on the back and performing any exercises that lift one or both legs, the hip flexors will be involved in the work. Never lift both straight legs off the floor or lower them at the same time as this can place tremendous strain on the lower back, even if the hands are underneath the buttocks or legs are bent.

F. Breathing

Breathing is especially important while performing abdominal exercises. Exhale while contracting the abdominals at the point of finishing your greatest exertion. For example: exhale as you sit up and inhale on the downward movement.

G. Variety

Vary your abdominal exercises. Exercises that include changing the position of the arms and legs, e.g., bent into the chest, lifted vertically in the air, elbow to knee twists or reverse curls, will work the abdominal muscles effectively and isolate these muscle groups without the use of momentum. While adding variety is important, performing only exercises that involve both torso and leg action will not isolate the abdominal muscles without using the hip flexors. A balanced combination of exercise variations that include exercises which stabilize the lower torso, as well as adding movement, is most beneficial.

H. Standing Abdominal Exercises

While exercises in a standing position, e.g., twisting or rotation, can be performed, these exercises do not effectively isolate the abdominal muscles against gravitational force.

While standing abdominal exercises may be utilized if proper standing alignment is followed, it is more advantageous to perform abdominal exercises in the supine position.

I. Common Problems

- arching the lower back
- arching the rib cage
- using neck motion only
- unsupported head
- using momentum
- not bringing shoulders and upper torso off the floor
- when breathing, pushing the abdominal muscles out
- rolling off the hips when performing rotation exercises
- using only elbow movement without torso twist for rotation
- throwing the legs too far toward head on a reverse curl

XII. Cool-Down Stretches

A. Purpose

To increase joint flexibility, relaxation and potential for reducing metabolic waste accumulated in the muscles from strengthening activities.

B. Time

Approximately 4-6 minutes at the very end of class is recommended.

C. Stretching

Follow the same guidelines as outlined for stretches at the beginning of class (see section V.C of this chapter). Static stretching is the most effective at the end of your class when the muscles are warm and prepared to stretch a little further. Now is the time to work on increasing flexibility, holding stretches a little longer (a minimum of 20 seconds) without bouncing, stretching a little further as the muscle relaxes.

D. Muscle Groups

Stretch all major muscle groups that were used during the workout, especially calves, hamstrings and quadriceps. Stretches for the back and upper torso should also be included. Include exercises that will balance muscle groups and improve posture and body alignment. It is not necessary to follow a particular exercise order as long as all major muscle groups are included.

E. Position

Final cool-down stretches can be performed in any position, e.g., lying, kneeling, sitting or standing, as long as correct body alignment is utilized so appropriate stretch techniques can be applied to the muscle that is being stretched.

1. Stretching the hamstrings when in an upright sitting position may be difficult for individuals with inflexible hamstrings and/or weak torso strength. Modify this stretch by bending one knee and stretching one leg at a time, or lie supine and stretch one hamstring at a time.

2. In a sitting position, legs should not be straddled to an extreme, but only to shoulder width or slightly more so the angle of toe to shoulder forms a diagonal line. The adductors can be sufficiently stretched without flexing forward from the hips. This position may be painful or uncomfortable for individuals with uneven hips, weak hip rotators, inflexible hamstrings or weak torso strength. Modify this stretch in any of these cases by bending one knee and stretching one leg at a time.

   a. If stretching forward from the hips, hands should be in a supporting position on the floor so the stretch forward is hip flexion, not bending from the waist in such a way that the upper torso collapses.

   b. If stretching laterally, the torso should also be supported by placing one hand on the floor to the front or side so the torso does not collapse.

   c. Placing elbows or chest on the floor to increase the degree of inner thigh stretch may stress the lumbar/sacral region. A safer alternative would be supine, knees bent with hands gently resisting outward on inner thighs.

F. Breathing

Inhale as you begin the stretch, then simultaneously stretch and relax the muscle as you exhale.

G. Exercises to Avoid

1. Don't do the "plow" as this position could cause injury to the neck. The vertebrae and discs in the cervical area were not designed to withstand this type of pressure. Modify with both knees into chest.

2. Don't do the "hurdler's stretch" as it places extreme tension on the medial ligaments of the knee. Modify with the inverted hurdler's stretch.

3. Don't do the "cobra" as this position hyperextends the lumbar spine, placing stress on the discs and connective tissue as well as hyperextending the elbows. Modify to the forearm-supported cobra position.

XIII. Final Heart Rate

A. Purpose

To determine if heart rate has sufficiently returned to normal pre-exercise range.

B. When to Take Heart Rate

Heart rate should be taken as static stretches are finished and class members prepare to leave.

C. Heart Rate

Again, the recovery heart rate equals 60% of estimated maximum heart rate (220 minus age, multiplied by .6) or less. If not below this level, the individual was probably exercising too intensely and should work at a less vigorous level during the next class. Cool-down stretches should be continued until heart rate is lowered.

D. Saunas and Hot Tubs

Saunas, hot tubs and even hot showers should be avoided immediately following exercise. The heat causes the blood vessels to dilate and this, along with the fact that the blood tends to be pooled in the extremities following vigorous exercise, causes the heart and brain to receive less blood and can cause overheating.

E. Hydration and Rehydration

Overheating can be a serious problem and special precautions should be taken, particularly in hot weather. Individuals should be advised to hydrate before, during and after exercise in order to replenish necessary body fluids and to maintain electrolyte balance. For every 20 minutes of exercise, allow 3 ounces of water. Salt tablets are not necessary unless involved in heavy endurance events, and even then should not be taken without consulting a sports physician or nutritionist. Deliberate dehydration by wearing heavy, rubberized clothes to induce profuse sweating is not recommended. The resulting weight loss is temporary and the weight will be regained through appropriate hydration. The practice of deliberate dehydration is very dangerous as it can cause death or brain damage due to very high body temperatures.

Part II

Specialty Populations

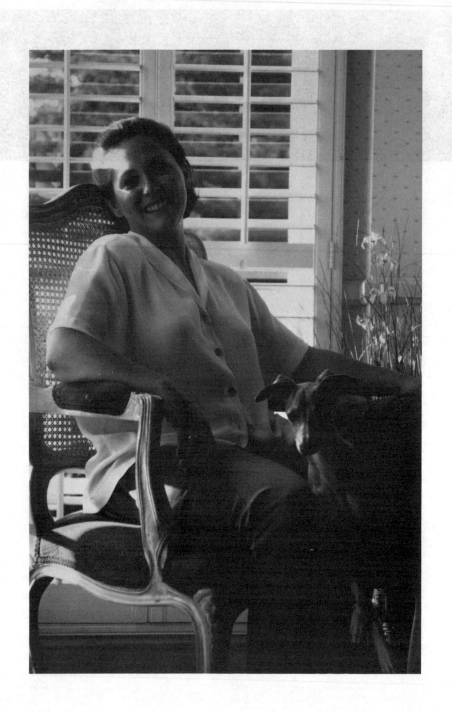

STANDARDS AND GUIDELINES

of the

Aerobics and Fitness Association of America

for the

Overweight Participant

I. Fitness for the Large-Size Exerciser—Program Justification

(Large-size exerciser may be defined as an individual who is overweight and/or overfat)

There are two primary goals for beginning and continuing a regular exercise program. The first is to maintain or improve the health of the body. The second is to gain enjoyment from the experience of moving the body in a pleasurable way. Historically, large-size individuals have not felt welcomed by the fitness industry, so only a limited number of them have been able to enjoy either of these benefits.

Many instructors have lacked the knowledge and confidence to provide safe and effective fitness programs for large-size exercisers. Coupled with the intimidation and anxiety felt by many large people when they begin an exercise program, the number of fitness programs suited to meet the needs of this special population has been small. But a growing number of large men and women are now claiming their rightful space in fitness facilities, and they are demanding knowledgeable and unbiased instructors of all sizes to be at their sides for education and support. These Standards and Guidelines are provided for instructors who are willing to meet that challenge.

II. Fat Bias

A. Societal Bias

The bias against fat people in our society is so pervasive that very few people can be bias-free without conscious effort. The degradation that fat people are subjected to by themselves and others does not create a self-image conducive to health enhancement.

B. The Instructor

It is essential that instructors choosing to work with large individuals address their own fat bias. Only then will they be able to see how their bias gets in the way of successful communication with their participants. The way instructors talk about their own bodies; their

39

fears concerning being fat; their desire to make everyone thin; the types of jokes they tell—these are all behaviors they can examine to increase awareness of and manage their own bias.

C. The Health Club Environment

The posters, graphics, instructor exercisewear, books and magazines present in many health clubs and studios often continue the adoration of the thin, ultra-fit physique. Fitness facilities should be aware that these images do not necessarily motivate all participants, particularly those whose bodies have already demonstrated an inability to conform to this thinner ideal. Showcasing images that reflect healthy people of all sizes and shapes will make the health club atmosphere more comfortable for large participants and will demonstrate a recognition of the true meaning of health.

III. Application

These Guidelines have been formulated to acquaint fitness instructors with the unique needs of large-size exercisers. Because there is such a large range of body shapes and sizes, no one rule necessarily applies to all large people. Also, because many large people are involved in a variety of sports and fitness activities, there is no intended implication that all large people are unfit.

These Guidelines are designed to meet the needs of the average healthy large person participating in an aerobic exercise class. Obviously, personal fitness trainers and instructors teaching classes of only large-size individuals will be able to implement these recommendations to the greatest extent. While guidelines are not provided in this chapter for step classes, weighted workouts, water exercise, exercise equipment, sports, etc., these are all viable options for large individuals. Use these Guidelines in conjunction with the "Basic Standards and Guidelines of the Aerobics and Fitness Association of America."

IV. Benefits of Consistent Exercise

The following lists of benefits of regular exercise are well-documented. Keep in mind that the physiological and musculoskeletal benefits are long-term and, therefore, may be less motivating than the psychosocial benefits. Placing the initial focus of exercise programs on science and education may deprive individuals of the most valuable ingredient to long-term adherence—pleasure.

A. Physiological Benefits of Exercise

1. Increased aerobic capacity

2. Decreased resting heart rate

3. Decreased blood pressure

4. Reduced serum cholesterol and triglycerides

5. Improved body composition

6. Improved hormonal function

B. Musculoskeletal Benefits of Exercise

1. Increased muscle strength and endurance

2. Increased muscle mass

3. Increased range of motion

4. Improved balance

5. Improved joint stability

6. Improved flexibility

C. Psychosocial Benefits of Exercise

1. Increased energy

2. Enhanced self-esteem and feelings of well-being

3. Increased feelings of self-efficacy

4. Opportunity for shared activity with family and friends

5. Improved sleep

6. Increased self-confidence and body-esteem

V. Participant Screening

A. Medical Clearance

It is discriminatory to require a medical clearance for participation based solely on the size of the individual. Every person beginning an exercise program, regardless of size, should complete a risk factor profile. The fitness instructor should follow the guidelines for medical clearance as outlined in "Basic Exercise Standards and Guidelines," section IV.A.

The primary responsibility for each individual's overall health management should lie with that person and his/her physician. In the case of a participant with health risk factors, a close alliance between the fitness instructor and the participant's physician is strongly recommended.

B. Fitness Evaluation and Testing

The administration of any kind of fitness testing, including strength, flexibility, body composition and cardiovascular endurance, unless specifically recommended by a physician, should be optional for the participant. While the results of these tests may provide motivation for some people, they may have just the opposite effect on others. The tests may take some people to the limits of their fitness abilities before they even begin, setting up a situation in which a person feels he/she must "pass" in order to participate. The instructor's primary goal should be to get participants moving as soon and as safely as possible. Fitness testing may be just one more barrier between the participant and an exercise regimen.

VI. Training Principles and Guidelines

The factors that need to be taken into consideration when personalizing an exercise program for large individuals are their: size, strength, flexibility, orthopedic limitations and health status, including the presence (if applicable) of risk factors. The participant's time schedule, exercise preferences, exercise history and goals must also be considered.

A. The Role of the Instructor as Lifestyle Educator

1. When guiding others through the process of a healthy lifestyle change, the instructor assumes many roles: facilitator, coach, educator and role model. Large-size individuals are no different than anyone else in their need to be treated with respect and to be heard. Instructors must have an understanding of the process of change and the various ways their participants will go through that process. Instructors should also realize that their most important responsibility, outside of teaching a safe and effective class, is to listen, not talk.

2. The lifestyle educator has perhaps the greatest impact on motivating the large participant to adopt healthy habits. Among other things, instructors should be able to:

    *   Maintain a professional manner that encompasses an unprejudiced and non-judgmental attitude toward their participants.

    *   Recognize individual differences in fitness and health levels.

    *   Act as a role model showing exercise as *iust one part* of a balanced mind, body and spirit.

    *   Show sincere interest in each participant and develop a rapport that leads to a relationship built on trust.

    *   Identify participants who need more support or more personalized attention.

    *   Show sensitivity, compassion and patience with every participant.

    *   Adapt exercise programs to meet individual needs.

    *   Teach proper technique, alignment and posture.

    *   Educate the participants as to which exercises increase strength, improve cardiorespiratory function, reduce body fat or increase flexibility.

    *   Impart a positive attitude toward exercise.

    *   Offer non-diet methods for changing eating behavior.

B. Goal Setting

Historically, large individuals have either been encouraged to lose weight before beginning an exercise program or their success with exercise has been linked so closely with weight loss that success with exercise seemed unachievable. When goal setting with large-size participants, instructors should not assume that weight loss is the desired goal. The instructor should ask what each participant's goals are, provide education as to the realistic nature of the goals and offer support for whatever the participant's chosen goals are. The instructor must be able to help the client differentiate between exercise and eating behavior goals, so that success with one is not dependent on success with the other.

C. Intensity/Duration

1. Research indicates that exercise training at a moderate intensity (55-70% of estimated maximum heart rate) for a long duration (minimum of 20 minutes) is optimal for health. The revised Borg Scale of Perceived Exertion is the recommended method for determining and monitoring the intensity of exercise for large individuals. Using this method, a recommended intensity level is **moderate to somewhat hard.**

The Borg Scale of Perceived Exertion

0	Nothing
.5	Extremely light
1	Very light
2	Light
3	Moderate
4	Somewhat hard
5	Heavy
6	
7	Very heavy
8	
9	
10	Extremely heavy

(Source: Borg, G.A.V., "Psychophysical Bases of Perceived Exertion." *Medicine and Science in Sport and Exercise* 14 (1982): 377-87.)

2. The location of body mass directly affects the intensity of the exercise. For example, if there is a large amount of body mass in the torso and upper extremities, exercises with arms elevated will increase the workload of the performing muscles and the cardiorespiratory system. Likewise, if there is a large amount of body mass in the hips, buttocks and lower extremities, elevating the legs (e.g., marching, knee lifts, etc.) will increase the workload.

D. Frequency

An exercise frequency of at least three days per week is recommended. For beginners, exercise frequency of more than three days per week and duration in excess of more than 45 minutes per session seems to offer the participant little additional gain in aerobic capacity, and appears to greatly increase the incidence of orthopedic injury. Even with an understanding of the importance of these recommendations, most participants are still faced with the reality of limited free time. For this reason, the goal should be to begin adopting a more active lifestyle. To that end, five minutes of exercise once or twice a week at the start may be a more reasonable way to begin.

E. **Rate of Progression**

Exercise must be of sufficient duration, intensity and frequency to create a training effect. This training effect will usually allow participants to increase their workload gradually over time. According to Blair and colleagues, research suggests that moderate levels of exercise can produce profound health changes. So there is no reason to push participants beyond their comfort level. Each participant's exercise program should be evaluated and adjusted accordingly.

F. **Body Alignment/Posture/Muscle Balancing**

See "Basic Exercise Standards and Guidelines," section I.D-E. In addition, the instructor should be particularly aware that sedentary individuals often lack the body awareness necessary for maintaining proper alignment when exercising. Common misalignments that may be obvious to the instructor on a thin person may not be as apparent on a larger person. One common misalignment in large individuals is the tibial vagus posture, also known as "knock-knee," in which the tibia follows a line that goes outward from its proximal to its distal end. Instructors should educate their participants on proper alignment while remaining aware of additional stresses that occur on joints with misalignment.

G. **Speed of Movement**

1. Body mass may affect joint range of motion as well as the ability of arms and legs to maneuver safely through rapid movement. All movement, including stretching, strengthening and cardiovascular conditioning should be performed with control. Rapid movements that utilize momentum should be avoided, as the additional body weight may place a physiological stress on the muscles and joints similar to a weighted workout.

2. Speed of movement has a direct impact on the intensity of the exercise. As heart rate should be carefully controlled, the speed of any movement should directly correlate with the size, shape, fitness level and exercise experience of the individual.

3. At least initially, not all large individuals will be comfortable moving from a standing position to the floor. Options should always be made available to perform the floor exercises in a standing or seated position. If moving to the floor, extra time should be allowed for transition from a floor-to-standing position or vice versa. Raising or lowering the large body should be accomplished slowly and carefully to avoid injury and reduce anxiety.

H. **Breathing**

1. Breathing should follow a consistent, rhythmic pattern throughout the class to avoid an increase in blood pressure. Inspire and expire through the nose and mouth in a relaxed fashion, always exhaling on the exertion.

2. Holding one's breath is a common problem with large exercisers, as moving or lifting additional body weight often requires extra effort. The instructor should avoid exercises that cause compression of the chest cavity (e.g., extreme forward flexion to stretch the buttocks/hamstrings) or may cause breathing problems.

3. Dyspnea (shortness of breath) and hypernea (rapid breathing), common with entry-level exercisers, may not only provoke fear and anxiety, but may also be caused by these emotions. Dyspnea and hypernea usually lessen or disappear over time.

4. Rapid heart rate, as it occurs in cardiovascular training, may be physically and emotionally uncomfortable for individuals who are experiencing it for the first time. Given the fact that most large individuals have been educated to believe they are candidates for a heart attack, the anxiety is easily understandable. The instructor should act as educator and compassionate coach in these circumstances.

I. Exercise Danger Signs

Know the Exercise Danger Signs as outlined in "Basic Exercise Standards and Guidelines," section III.A. As part of the pre-class instruction, participants should be advised to inform the instructor of any pain or discomfort they may experience during class. When working with entry-level exercisers, pay special attention to observing outward signs of physical distress and fatigue that could possibly lead to a more serious condition or injury.

J. Music

Research into the effects of music on exercise performance reveals energy expenditure generally increases while perceived exertion generally decreases when music accompanies exercise. The results indicate that music may act as a stimulus that takes the mind away from the physical manifestations of exercise. This may have both a positive and negative influence on the exerciser. On the positive side, music takes participants' minds off exercise, thereby allowing them to accomplish more of the workload with less awareness of discomfort or fatigue. On the negative side, this lessened awareness may cause participants to exercise too strenuously, making them more prone to injury or exceeding their recommended intensity levels. The fitness instructor, recognizing the value of music as a motivating factor, should be watchful of any indicators that a participant is overexercising as a result of involvement with the music.

K. Special Exercise Considerations

Keep in mind that an entry-level exerciser may initially have difficulty meeting the minimums of exercise frequency, intensity and duration. The exercise training minimums should be incorporated only when the participant is physically able to accomplish them without injury, abnormally elevated heart rate or undue muscle fatigue. To avoid these anxiety-producing consequences of overexercise, a low-intensity interval training program may be an option for certain individuals as it allows the instructor to alternate exercises which sustain a higher heart rate with those that do not. Balance the participants' fitness levels with their comfort levels.

VII. Class Format

A. Sequence

See "Basic Exercise Standards and Guidelines," section II.

Sequence takes on greater importance with large exercisers as transitioning from floor to standing is not always easily accomplished. It may be preferable in some cases to conduct the entire class in a standing or chair-seated position to avoid the strain of lifting and lowering the body to the floor. If floorwork is included, avoid a great deal of floor-to-standing transitions.

B. Types of Movement

1. Aerobic exercise, which utilizes the large muscle groups and is rhythmical in nature, benefits the cardiovascular system and improves body composition. Because muscle strengthening exercises increase lean body mass, they have a positive effect on body composition profiles. The large skeletal muscles are avid calorie consumers, so an increase in muscle mass has an impact on overall energy expenditure. Cardiovascular conditioning exercises contribute to the maintenance of lean tissue while strengthening exercises build lean tissue.

2. Physical limitations for large exercisers are not necessarily different from those of thin people, nor are large exercisers more prone to injury in class. Orthopedic problems the fitness instructor may encounter in participants include arthritis, as well as lower back, hip, knee and ankle joint discomfort. In the presence of pain or discomfort, weight-bearing activities may be alternated with non-weight-bearing activities as a method of avoiding stress on the joints.

3. Research shows that while large exercisers usually have good motor coordination, their additional weight can make balance a limiting factor in exercise performance, comfort and enjoyment. The class format should, therefore, include exercises that improve body awareness and balance. A common concern among large people is the fear of falling down during exercise. This often comes from a lack of trust that they can move their large bodies safely. These fears should dissipate over time. In the meantime, supported balance exercises (e.g., using a wall or ballet barre) and kinesthetic awareness exercises (e.g., touching the biceps as they contract) may help to build confidence and allay fears.

VIII. Overview of Exercise for Large-Size Individuals

A. For both psychological and physiological reasons, attending an exercise class may be a stressful experience for the large person who is new to exercise. The instructor should be cognizant of this and should try, **by listening and reassuring, to alleviate as much stress as possible.**

B. The fitness instructor should recognize that participation in an exercise program is often the first step toward a more comprehensive lifestyle change. The instructor should **be responsive to the participant's need for support and encouragement.** The instructor should be prepared to refer the participant to reputable professionals in other health professions (e.g., nutrition, stress management, etc.).

C. The instructor should give clear, concise instructions in every class for each exercise. Describe the exercises "generically" (e.g., "Reach *toward* your feet" rather than "Hold onto your feet") to accommodate the variety of strength and flexibility levels in the class.

D. In the initial stages of training, exercises that are easily accomplished may be preferable to those that offer a challenge. Feelings of inadequacy are thereby avoided and the participant's confidence in his/her ability to succeed in this endeavor begins to build at the outset.

E. Entry-level exercisers may prefer exercises that are repetitive over a period of time so they are able to notice improvements in coordination, strength, flexibility and confidence immediately.

F. Not all exercises are recommended for the large exerciser as some movements may be awkward to perform or inappropriate for the larger body size or shape. **Exercise selection should be based on the instructor's knowledge of each class participant.**

G. Stretch out more often than usual. This helps to dispel any associations participants may make between exercise and discomfort. It also provides a pertinent break between more strenuous exercises.

IX. Pre-Class Instruction

A. Pre-class Procedures

See "Basic Exercise Standards and Guidelines," section IV.

B. Participant Expectations of an Exercise Program

A major factor for maintaining long-term adherence (6 months or longer) in an exercise program is a realistic set of expectations. External physical results usually follow long after internal physiological and psychological results. To avoid discouragement with exercise, it is incumbent on the instructor to educate the large exerciser concerning the expected results of exercise and a realistic time frame for seeing or feeling the manifestations of these results. While research cannot yet confirm exact times or results, a fair analysis of data indicates that the first conditioning effects may be visible 6 to 12 weeks into a consistent exercise program. It may be of more importance to large participants to focus on their ability to move and breathe with greater ease as well as the actions they've been taking to accomplish that ability. They should also be encouraged to focus on the pleasure of movement. The instructor should NOT pitch exercise as just another means of quick weight loss because it will encourage participants to adopt a diet mentality around exercise (e.g., all-or-nothing thinking; feelings of failure; a need to be thin in order to succeed; attempts to be perfect; etc.).

C. Skin Abrasions

Fitness instructors should be aware that some large exercisers may experience skin irritation due to chafing. Participants should be advised to closely monitor areas where skin irritation might occur (e.g., inside of thighs). If the problem is chronic, medical attention should be sought.

D. Attire

1. The importance of wearing shoes appropriate to the activity is now well understood. This is especially true for large exercisers who also depend on shoes for added stability. Additional factors affecting shoe selection may include adequate ventilation and shoe width. Participants should be advised that their shoes are likely to wear out faster and should be replaced more often.

2. Many large women are uncomfortable wearing revealing exercise clothes. Inappropriate workout clothes, however, are uncomfortable and may affect exercise performance by causing heat stress (e.g., polyester fabrics that don't breathe or long-sleeved sweats that are too warm). There is finally a greater selection of workout clothes available for large exercisers. A list of stores and catalogues with exercisewear for large men and women should be made available to every new large participant. Participants should be encouraged to wear fabrics that breathe (e.g., cotton). Choice of attire should also reflect environment and temperature/humidity.

X. Warm-Up

A. See "Basic Exercise Standards and Guidelines," section V.

B. Special Considerations

1. Psychological preparation should be incorporated into the warm-up by means of gradual movements and verbal motivation from the instructor.

2. Emphasis should be placed on dynamic movements that utilize the large muscle groups through their full range of motion.

3. Special attention should be given to properly preparing the lower back, and shoulder, hip, knee and ankle joints for the more vigorous exercises to follow.

4. Include exercises which improve body awareness and balance. For participants who are just beginning exercise training, utilize support for the balancing exercises.

C. Precautions

1. Select a speed of movement that allows participants to achieve full range of motion without momentum.

2. Supported forward flexion should not compress the chest or abdominal area to the point that it inhibits breathing.

3. If there is a greater amount of body mass in the medial deltoid area, do not force the arm toward the ear as it may lead to dizziness.

4. Warm-up should be accomplished in a standing or chair-seated position.

5. Exercise selection should be congruent with the fitness level of the participants.

6. Elbow and knee joint hyperextension should be avoided.

XI. Cardiovascular Conditioning

A. See "Basic Exercise Standards and Guidelines," section VI.A-H.

B. Special Considerations

1. Low-impact aerobics is the recommended method for attaining cardiovascular conditioning. Low-impact aerobics significantly lessens the amount of stress normally associated with high-impact aerobics.

2. Start slowly and gradually increase the intensity and range of motion of the movements. Movements should be controlled, resistive and non-ballistic.

3. Arm and leg elevation should be varied to control heart rate and reduce the stress on joints.

4. Leg elevation should directly correlate to the flexibility, strength and fitness level of the individual.

5. Combination moves requiring coordination of both arms and legs should be entered into slowly, starting with either the arms or the legs and then adding the other in order to build in positive experiences with movement.

C. Precautions

1. Entry-level exercisers often have difficulty pacing themselves. Watch for signs of overexertion.

2. Do not include movements which rely strictly on momentum for execution.

3. High-impact aerobics is inappropriate for most large exercisers. Certain large people who have been participating in a consistent exercise program of walking or low-impact aerobics, and are free of orthopedic problems, may gradually begin a high-impact aerobics program.

4. Some lateral movements may be difficult for certain large participants. Always offer a side-step alternative.

5. Avoid movements that require a quick turn unless the movement is executed at such a slow speed that large participants will not risk torqueing their knees or ankles to complete it.

6. Avoid movements that may result in slipping, twisting the ankles or hyperextending the joints.

XII. Post-Aerobic Cool-Down

A. See "Basic Exercise Standards and Guidelines," section VII.A-D.

B. Special Considerations

For entry-level exercisers, a longer cool-down is recommended.

C. Precautions

Use the Borg Scale of Perceived Exertion (see section VI.C of this chapter) to monitor the participant's intensity level following the cool-down period. If the participant still identifies an intensity of "moderate" or higher, he/she should be advised to work at a lower intensity.

XIII. Upper Body Strengthening Exercises

A. See "Basic Exercise Standards and Guidelines," section VIII.

B. Special Considerations

1. Weakness in the upper body is common in inactive large participants, especially women, due to poorly developed and atrophied muscles.
2. Movements should be resistive, smooth, controlled and slow enough to allow for complete extension.
3. Free weights (or other resistive equipment) may be used to bring about a more rapid muscular strength response. Free weights should only be introduced once the participant is able to complete a non-weighted workout with controlled contraction and without undue fatigue. Utilization of free weights should begin with the lowest weight, adding additional weight only when the participant is able to complete 16 repetitions in the same range of motion without undue fatigue.
4. The decision to incorporate push-ups should be based on the participant's strength and orthopedic limitations, as push-ups on the floor increase stress on the shoulders and wrists. Weight-supported modifications (e.g., doing push-ups against the wall from a standing position) lessen the stress and may be more appropriate in the initial stages of training.

C. Precautions

1. When there is a greater amount of body mass in the arms, leverage is the key factor in the safe and effective performance of upper body work. Large individuals should be instructed to perform short lever movements if fatigue sets in or if momentum begins to replace slow, resistive movement.

2. If standing, elbow and knee joints should not be hyperextended.

3. Vary the arm elevation, lever length and range of motion to avoid early fatigue and stress on the joints.

XIV. Legs, Hips and Buttocks Strengthening Exercises

A. See "Basic Exercise Standards and Guidelines," section IX.

B. Special Considerations

1. In many cases, the lower body, excluding the abdomen, has undergone a slow, progressive strength adaptation to accommodate a larger individual's increased body weight. The instructor may, therefore, see greater muscular strength and endurance in the performance of lower body exercises.

2. For hip abduction in the side-lying position, the upper body should be totally supported in a comfortable position. Depending on body mass distribution, there are three positions to choose from: the torso is lying fully extended on the floor; the torso is raised up on one elbow with the head supported by the hand; or the torso is raised up on one elbow with the supporting hand placed flat on the floor. The instructor should educate the participants as to the position options and guide them toward choosing the most comfortable position in which they can also maintain alignment.

3. It is difficult to achieve significant range of motion performing hip adduction in the side-lying position with the top leg in front if there is great body mass in the inner thigh area. An alternate position is with the foot of the top leg placed behind the working leg, as long as there is no torque on the knee or ankle and body mass in the buttocks can support the spine.

4. During the initial stages of training, the all-fours position for gluteals and hamstrings should be performed with the upper body resting on the elbows rather than on the hands. This position improves balance, decreases the amount of weight that needs to be supported and reduces the risk of spinal hyperextension due to the pull of gravity.

5. Hip adduction in the supine position should be performed with both feet placed on the floor if: (a) a greater amount of body mass in the hips, buttocks and lower extremities makes it difficult to keep the back on the floor or (b) a lack of strength makes it difficult to keep both elevated legs at a 90-degree angle to the body.

6. Standing leg lifts to strengthen quadriceps should be performed with support (e.g., wall, ballet barre, etc.).

C. Precautions

1. Squats and lunges are inappropriate quadriceps strengthening exercises for large individuals due to the stress they place on the knees.

51

2. When there is a greater amount of body mass in the lower body, leverage is the key factor in the safe and effective performance of lower body work for large individuals.

Participants should be instructed to work with a short lever if fatigue sets in or if momentum begins to replace slow, resistive movement.

XV. Abdominal Strengthening Exercises

A. See "Basic Exercise Standards and Guidelines," section XI.

B. **Special Considerations**

1. Large individuals with considerable abdominal mass are likely to have great difficulty performing effective abdominal exercises in the supine position due to limited range of motion and an increased workload. The extra layers of fat make it nearly impossible to feel the muscles contracting. The instructor should teach body awareness and emphasize contraction rather than lifting in the initial stages of exercise training.

2. The decision to incorporate sit-ups in the supine position should be based on the participant's strength and the presence of abdominal mass that might limit range of motion. Weight-supported modifications (e.g., holding onto a towel wrapped behind the legs to assist with a lift in the supine position) may be appropriate.

3. Standing abdominal exercises are an ideal modification for participants who choose not to perform abdominal strengthening in the supine position. There are two recommended exercises: spinal rotation and the standing crunch. Both exercises should be performed slowly, with conscious resistive contraction.

4. Abdominal strengthening exercises may be performed in the all-fours position on hands and knees. Participants should be instructed to contract the abdominals up toward the spine or ceiling and then relax them without allowing the spine to lose alignment on the relaxation phase.

C. **Precautions**

1. Breathing is especially important when performing abdominal exercises. As supine abdominal work involves, by its nature, a degree of compression to the chest cavity, care should be taken to move slowly enough so breathing is not inhibited. Holding one's breath is common among large participants during abdominal strengthening. The instructor should make frequent reminders to exhale on the exertion.

2. The participant should be advised not to rely on momentum to lift the shoulders off the floor. Additionally, all movement should be slow enough that the participant is able to physically identify a "start" and "stop" to each curl-up.

3. Support for the head should be incorporated on an individual basis as needed. The flexibility of the participant may not allow for a comfortable hands-behind-the-head position. If additional support is needed, offer the participant a pillow or folded towel to place under his/her head to prevent it from falling out of alignment.

XVI. Cool-Down Stretches/Final Heart Rate

A. See "Basic Exercise Standards and Guidelines," sections XII-XIII.

B. Special Considerations

1. Many sedentary large individuals experience chronic back discomfort. Including stretches for the upper and lower back may help relieve some of this discomfort, while providing participants with the tools for alleviating discomfort on their own. This process also helps the participant associate exercise with good feelings, both physically and emotionally.

2. Participants with flexibility limitations due to greater abdominal or lower body mass may enhance their stretches with the use of props (e.g., holding on to a towel wrapped around the foot for a supine hamstring stretch).

C. Precaution

Exercise selection should take into consideration the flexibility and location of body mass of each class participant. The instructor should be prepared to offer modifications for all stretches.

References

Brownell, K.D., & Foreyt, J.P. (Eds.) (1986). *Handbook of eating disorders: Physiology, psychology, and treatment of obesity, anorexia and bulimia*. New York: Basic Books.

Denke, M.A., Sempos, C.T., & Grundy, S.M. (1993). Excess body weight: An underrecognized contributor to high blood cholesterol levels in white american men. *Archives of Internal Medicine*, 153, 1093-1103.

Ducimetiere, P., & Richard, J.L. (1989). The relationship between subsets of anthropometric upper versus lower body measurements and coronary heart disease risk in middle-aged men. The Paris Prospective Study. *International Journal of Obesity*, 13: 111-12.

Health implications of obesity. (February 11-13, 1985). *Annals of Internal Medicine*, 103: 981-1077.

Hubert, H.B., Feinleib, M., McNamara, P.M., et al (1983). Obesity as an independent risk factor for cardiovascular disease: A 26-year follow-up of participants in the framingham study. *Circulation*, 67: 968-77.

Kannel, W.B., Brand, N., Skinner, J.J., Dawber, T.R., & McNamara, P.M. (1967). The relation of adiposity to blood pressure and development of hypertension. The Framingham Study. *Annals of Internal Medicine*, 67: 48-59.

Keesey, R.E. (1986). A set-point theory of obesity. In K.D. Brownell and J.P. Foreyt (Eds.), *Handbook of eating disorders: Physiology, psychology and treatment of obesity, anorexia and bulimia*. New York: Basic Books.

Kopelman, P.G., Apps, M.LC., Cope, T., Ingram, D.A., Empey, D.W., & Evans, S.J. (1986). Nocturnal hypoxia and sleep apnoea in asymptomatic obese men. *International Journal of Obesity*, 10: 211-17.

Maclure, K.M., Hayes, K.C., Colditz, G.A., Stampfer, J.J., Speizer, F.E., & Willett, W.C. (1989). Weight, diet, and the risk of symptomatic gallstones in middle-aged women. *New England Journal of Medicine*, 321: 563-9.

MacMahon, S.W., Blacket, R.B., Macdonald, G.J., & Hall, W. (1984). Obesity, alcohol consumption and blood pressure in australian men and women. The National Heart Foundation of Australia Risk Factor Prevalence Study. *Journal of Hpertension*, 2: 85-91.

Methods for voluntary weight loss and control: National institutes of health technology assessment conference. (1993). *Annals of Internal Medicine*, 119: 7.

Najjar, M.F., & Rowland, M. (October,1 1987). Anthropometric reference data and prevalence of overweight, United States, 1976-80. *Vital and Health Statistics*. Series 11, No. 238. DHHS Pub. No. (PHS) 87-1688. Public Health Service, Washington, D.C.: U.S. Government Printing Office.

National institutes of health consensus development conference statement. *Health Implications of Obesity*.

Pollock, M.L., & Wilmore, J.H. (1990). *Exercise in health and disease*. Philadelphia: W.B. Saunders Co.

Rimm, A.A., Werner, L.H., Yserloo, B.V., & Bernstein, R.A. (1975). Relationship of obesity and disease in 73,532 weight-conscious women. *Public Health Reports*, 90, 44-54.

Van Itallie, T.B. (1985). Health implications of overweight and obesity in the United States. *Annals of Internal Medicine*, 103: 983-8.

Welham, W.C., & Behnke, A.R. (1942). The specific gravity of healthy men: Body weight divided by volume and other physical characteristics of exceptional athletes and of naval personnel. *Journal of the American Medical Association*, 118: 498-501.

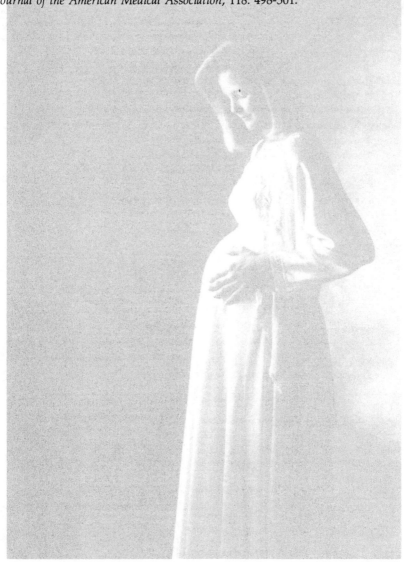

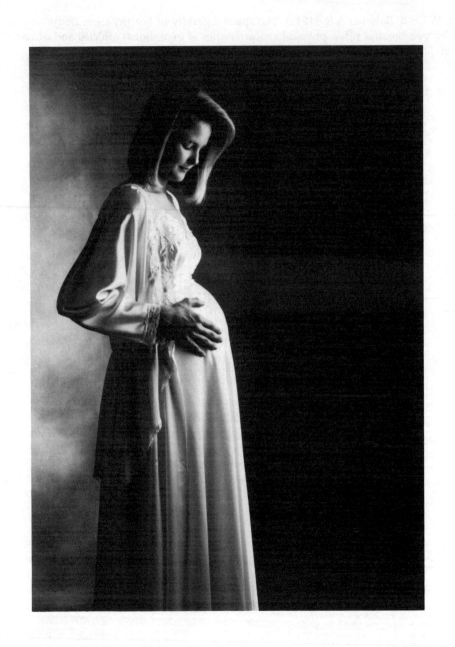

STANDARDS AND GUIDELINES

of the
Aerobics and Fitness Association of America
for

Prenatal Exercise

Objectives

Upon completion of this section, the participant will be able to:

1. List the benefits of prenatal exercise.

2. Demonstrate awareness of prenatal exercise.

3. List the importance of medical clearance for the expectant mother prior to participation in an exercise program.

4. Develop a safe exercise program for the prenatal exerciser.

Introduction

During the past 20 years, the United States has experienced a fitness revolution. Record numbers of people, spending millions of dollars, have sought the benefits of exercise. Coinciding with this upsurge of interest in keeping fit has been the increase in the number of women entering the workplace and pursuing careers. Consequently, many women in the 1990's now approach their pregnancies as they would a timeline for a special project at work. From conception through delivery, every step of the pregnancy is planned, for maximum returns—a healthy baby, an efficient delivery and a quick return to the pre-pregnancy body. A perceived determinant in achieving these goals is the health and fitness level of the mother-to-be. Many women today see exercise during pregnancy as an integral part of their prenatal program.

AFAA heartily supports this trend toward prenatal health and fitness. However, in most cases, today's expectant mother does not enter a prenatal exercise program that is based on firmly established standards. Stories passed down from generation to generation, some accurate, others full of fallacy, still influence the decisions many women make regarding prenatal care and exercise. Other more recent and respected sources of information are often confusing and ill-defined.

For health care and fitness professionals, this interest in prenatal exercise poses many questions such as: How much exercise is too much and what types of exercise are contraindicated? Very often, limitations and guidelines are not clear to students nor instructors. AFAA, through the research of many respected individuals in the fields of obstetrics, exercise physiology and fitness instruction, proposes the following Standards and Guidelines for safe and effective prenatal exercise.

These Guidelines are designed to be used in conjunction with the "Basic Exercise Standards and Guidelines of the Aerobics and Fitness Association of America."

I. Benefits of Prenatal Exercise

A. Physiological Benefits of Exercise

1. Increased aerobic capacity

2. Improved circulation

3. Improved digestion and elimination

4. Improved energy and endurance

5. More restful sleep

B. Musculoskeletal Benefits of Exercise

1. Improved muscular strength and endurance will increase muscular efficiency during labor and delivery

2. Increased range of motion

3. Improved balance

4. Improved muscle tone to support joints

5. Improved flexibility and mobility

6. Improved posture and possible prevention of permanent postural deviation and associated discomforts

7. Improved support of pelvic organs

C. Psychosocial Benefits of Exercise

1. Reduced tension, anxiety and fatigue

2. Enhanced feeling of well-being

3. Improved self-image

4. Opportunity for shared activity with family, friends and other pregnant women

5. Improved physical control over body increases confidence in an otherwise uncontrollable situation

6. Deep relaxation exercises assist in establishing a stronger conditioned response to control discomforts of labor

II. Participant Screening

A. Medical Clearance

All individuals beginning an exercise program should follow the guidelines for medical clearance as stated in "Basic Exercise Standards and Guidelines," section IV.A. Additionally, to avoid risk of injury to participants and litigative risk to instructors, attendance in your class should be limited to those with physician's written approval. The primary responsibility for the health management of the woman's pregnancy should lie with her physician. The decision of when to commence and when to cease an exercise program rests with the physician. A close alliance between the fitness instructor and the participant's physician is strongly recommended.

B. Health Risk Appraisal

It is important to evaluate an individual's level of fitness prior to commencement of an exercise program for the following reasons:

1. To determine the current level of physical fitness and overall health status.

2. To objectively evaluate an individual's response to exercise.

3. To determine an appropriate workload when individualizing an exercise regimen.

C. Role of Instructor in Health Screening Process

Only qualified specialists may assess the safety of exercise, administer an exercise stress test and write an exercise prescription for the prospective prenatal exercise class participant. The instructor should design an initial interview and health questionnaire that will reveal the information necessary to make sound recommendations for more extensive screening when it is apparently necessary.

It is again recommended that all class participants have written approval from their physician. A physician will have recently completed a thorough physical and health history on a prospective student and, therefore, will be most qualified to identify an appropriate level of exercise and any limitations. It should be noted that health histories taken by a physician may fail to reveal prior orthopedic problems and postural deviations. Due to the known added weight gain associated with pregnancy, evaluation of any orthopedic condition is important. Questions related to prior orthopedic or postural problems should be included in the questionnaire. Refer any questions to the woman's physician.

D. Exercise Contraindications

    1. Absolute Contraindications

        a. active myocardial disease

        b. congestive heart failure

        c. rheumatic heart disease (a classification of II and above)

        d. thrombophlebitis

        e. recent pulmonary embolism

        f. acute infectious disease

        g. at risk for premature labor, incompetent cervix

        h. multiple gestations

        i. uterine bleeding, ruptured membranes

        j. intrauterine growth retardation or macrosomia

        k. severe isoimmunization

        l. severe hypertensive disease

        m. no prenatal care

        n. suspected fetal distress

    2. Relative Contraindications

        a. essential hypertension

        b. anemia or other blood disorders

        c. thyroid disease

        d. diabetes mellitus

        e. breech presentation in last trimester

        f. excessive obesity, overweight or extreme underweight

III. Training Principles and Guidelines

A. Intensity

    1. Heart Rate

        a. Resting heart rate may increase as much as 10-15 bpm.

        b. Pregnant women reach maximum cardiac output at a lower level of work than non-pregnant women.

        c. A meta-analysis of the human research available has shown that women have exercised up to intensitites of 144 bpm for as long as 43 minutes with no ill effects on the fetus. Research beyond these levels is scant.

d. Exercise heart rate range should fall between 55% to 70% of age-predicted maximum heart rate. The more fit exerciser may exercise up to 75% of MHR, but neither fit nor unfit pregnant exercisers should exceed 144 bpm due to lack of research beyond this range.

e. The 1994 American College of Obstetrics and Gynecology (ACOG) guidelines give no specific restrictions for intensity for aerobic exercise, but emphasize the need to listen to one's own maternal symptoms, and stop exercising when fatigued. Due to the lack of body awareness of the unfit pregnant exerciser, AFAA still recommends the above guidelines for exercise intensity.

f. Heart rate is more variable in response to exercise.

    i. Check pulse every 4-5 minutes during peak activities.

    ii. Make sure that pulse is not sustained over training heart rate.

    iii. Use Karvonen formula to incorporate changes in resting heart rate (220 - age - resting heart rate x % [55 to 75] of estimated maximum heart rate range + resting heart rate = training heart rate).

2. Perceived Exertion

a. Best indicator of workload tolerance during both cardiovascular training and recovery.

b. Train at similar intensity (physiological strain), not same workload.

c. Train at the "somewhat hard" level on Borgs Scale of relative perceived exertion (RPE).

B. Duration

1. Class time should not exceed 1 hour and 15 minutes.

2. If student has been performing regular aerobic exercise for at least 6 months prior to pregnancy, she may continue her current program provided she is monitored by a physician and has no discomfort or danger signs. If current duration is maintained, the intensity should be reduced to the levels stated above. Exercising for periods longer than 45 minutes, however, carries a high risk of hypoglycemia and increased body temperature.

3. For the unfit pregnant student, cardiovascular training should gradually build up to, but not exceed, 20 to 30 minutes, including pre-aerobic phase through post-aerobic cool-down.

C. Frequency

Participants should exercise 3 to 4 times per week. More frequent training requires careful monitoring for signs of overtraining or complications of pregnancy. Regular prenatal care is recommended.

D. Rate of Progression

1. Pregnancy is a time to maintain fitness, not strive for dramatic improvements. As body weight increases, workload will normally decrease.

2. Beginning students may be able to increase workload slightly at start of program.

E. Posture and Alignment

Instructors should be aware a woman's center of gravity becomes displaced during pregnancy, and maintaining good posture and alignment becomes progressively more difficult.

1. Lordosis

    a. Enlarging uterus pulls center of gravity forward.
       i. center of gravity constantly changes.

       ii. risk of falling increases.

    b. Abdominal muscles lengthen and stretch. Back extensors and hip flexors shorten.
       i. focus on strengthening abdominals and stretching lower back.

       ii. overuse of hip flexors in kicks and knee lifts may aggravate lordosis.

2. Kyphosis

    a. Weight of enlarging breasts pulls shoulders forward; chin juts outward.

    b. Strong chest muscles are important to support increased weight of breasts. However, an individual must balance strengthening of pectoralis with trapezius, rhomboids and latissimus dorsi to avoid muscle and postural imbalance.

    c. "Chin jut" is the result of weak cervical spine flexors and shortened cervical spine extensors.

    d. Neck strengthening exercises such as dropping chin to chest while gently pressing upward on chin with the hand may be helpful.

3. Pelvic Tilt

    a. Students should follow the basic guidelines for body alignment found in "Basic Exercise Standards and Guidelines," section I.E.

    b. Additionally, pregnant students should be encouraged to tilt the pelvis (bottom of the pelvis forward) in all positions, e.g., sitting, standing and lying down, in order to counteract the postural misalignments outlined above. This may help maintain pelvic neutral alignment, ease associated discomfort, particularly in the lower back, and may help prevent permanent postural problems.

F. Breathing

Frequent feelings of dyspnea may be caused by the uterus crowding the diaphragm.

1. Breathing should follow a consistent rhythmic pattern throughout the class to avoid an increase in blood pressure. Inspire and expire through the nose and mouth in a relaxed fashion, always exhaling on the exertion. Reminders to breathe rhythmically should be made throughout the class.

2. Holding one's breath can elicit the Valsalva maneuver which can increase intra-abdominal pressure.

G. Danger Signs

1. Know the Exercise Danger Signs as outlined in "Basic Exercise Standards and Guidelines," section III.A, 2b.

2. Signs and symptoms indicating immediate cessation of exercise and referral to physician's care:

   a. pain of any kind—chest, head, back, pubic or hip

   b. uterine contractions (frequent at 20-minute intervals)

   c. vaginal bleeding, leaking of amniotic fluid

   d. dizziness, faintness

   e. shortness of breath

   f. palpitation, tachycardia

   g. persistent nausea and vomiting

   h. difficulty walking

   i. generalized edema

   j. decreased fetal activity

3. When working with pregnant exercisers, special attention must be paid to observing outward signs of physical distress and fatigue that could possibly lead to a more dangerous condition.

H. Music

Research into the effect of music on exercise performance reveals that energy expenditure generally increases while perceived exertion generally decreases when music accompanies exercise. The results may indicate that music acts as a stimulus that takes the mind away from the physical manifestations of exercise. Although enhancing the individual's enjoyment of exercise, this lessened awareness may cause a participant to exercise too strenuously, making her more prone to injury or exceeding her training heart rate. The fitness instructor should be observant of any indicators that a participant is over exercising as a result of involvement with the music.

1. Because of displaced center of gravity and resulting risk of imbalance and added weight, music should be slightly slower for the pregnant exerciser. This will decrease the tendency to move too quickly which can cause falling and other injury.

   a. During low-impact cardiovascular conditioning, music should not exceed 125 to 145 bpm.

   b. Music utilized for floorwork should stay in the 120 to 130 bpm range.

I. Additional Special Exercise Considerations

1. Hormonal Changes Affecting Joints

   a. Relaxin, estrogen, progesterone and elastin increase, causing softening of cartilage and relaxation of ligaments.

   b. Pelvic joints soften and widen, causing unstable pelvis and change in gait, especially in the third trimester.

   c. Potential for injury increases for joints and connective tissue.

      i. avoid excessive bouncing and jarring of joints especially for untrained women.

      ii. avoid stretching to maximum resistance.

      iii. avoid deep flexion of the knees.

2. Cardiovascular and Hemodynamic Changes

   a. Blood volume increases.

   b. Increased progesterone causes vasodilation to maintain normal arterial pressure.

      i. students may be more susceptible to postural hypotension.

   c. Venous pressure continues to rise gradually after the eighth week of pregnancy.

      i. increased risk of varicosities in legs, vulva and rectum.

      ii. avoid constrictive clothing or prolonged standing.

3. Carpal Tunnel Syndrome

   a. Water retention causes edema in ankles and wrists, reducing mobility.

   b. Edema compresses median nerves running through carpal in wrists.

   c. Symptoms may include tingling in thumb and index and middle fingers.

   d. Hyperflexion of wrists for prolonged periods may produce symptoms.

      i. exercise on all fours or wall push-ups involving weight-bearing wrist flexion may initiate symptoms in women with carpal tunnel syndrome.

4. Supine Hypotensive Syndrome

   a. Enlarging uterus may compress vena cava in supine position.

   b. Reduces venous return to heart and decreases cardiac output.

   c. Mother may become hypotensive.

      i. feels dizzy, lightheaded, nauseous, pale or flushed.

      ii. maternal symptoms will manifest before blood flow to placenta is critically decreased.

      iii. if symptomatic, roll to left side.

      iv. exercise in the supine position should not exceed three to four minutes.

      v. if consistently symptomatic or if restricted by physician, alternative exercises should be substituted.

   d. The American College of Obstetricians and Gynecologists recommends that an individual with symptoms of, or diagnosed with Supine Hypotensive Syndrome should not exercise in a supine position.

   e. Prolonged motionless standing has also been shown to significantly reduce cardiac output, and therefore should be avoided.

5. Leg Cramps

   a. Forceful or prolonged pointing of toes can initiate painful contraction of the calf muscle and should be avoided.

6. Hydration and Heat Loss

   a. Pregnant women are not as efficient as non-pregnant women at exchanging heat.

      i. pregnant women tend to store fat.

      ii. fat insulates and decreases heat loss.

      iii. core temperature increases.

   b. Sustained vigorous activity (20 to 30 minutes) increases body core temperature. Benefits of training include:

      i. partial acclimatization.

      ii. sweating occurs sooner.

      iii. lowering of core temperature.

   c. Fetus cannot dissipate heat as fast as the mother can—it must wait for a temperature gradient to occur.

   d. Hydration before, during and after exercise affects temperature.

      i. dehydration increases core temperature to dangerous levels.

      ii. dehydration has been known to precipitate premature labor.

      iii. encourage students to drink water before, during and after class despite concern with urinary frequency.

      iv. encourage students to monitor the color of their urine—a dark yellow color may indicate dehydration.

IV. Class Format

A. Sequence

See "Basic Exercise Standards and Guidelines," section II.A-B.

1. Additional Considerations for Pregnant Participants:

    a. Changing position from one exercise to another and getting up and down off of the floor takes additional time and effort.

    b. Performing specific muscular toning exercises prior to cardiovascular training may fatigue large muscle groups, rendering the aerobic segment difficult and possibly increasing risk of injury.

    c. Specific exercises for strengthening the pelvic floor should be added early in pregnancy.

        i. weight of uterus places tremendous downward pressure on pelvic floor.

        ii. weak muscles may cause stress, urinary incontinence, postnatal sexual dysfunction and uterine prolapse.

        iii. see section XV of this chapter for specific pelvic floor exercises.

B. Types of Movement

1. Because of painful pull on round ligaments, rapid twisting and directional changes should be avoided.

    a. Hips should face forward when performing lateral movements.

2. Displaced center of gravity increases risk of losing balance.

    a. Movements should be performed at a moderate pace which allows for careful transition from one direction to another.

3. Transitions and cueing for exercise or directional changes should be described well in advance.

    a. Always make sure that the upper body is supported and stable before moving.

    b. When moving from a sitting to a standing position:

        i. support body with hand on floor as weight is transferred to knee.

        ii. bring other foot forward.

        iii. support body weight on top of thigh when coming to a full standing position.

        iv. move feet right away.

        v. reverse procedure when moving from a standing to a sitting position.

c. When moving from a sitting to a lying position:

    i.   roll to the side onto the hip, walk the body down with hands, arms supporting upper body weight.

    ii. Reverse when moving from a position lying on the floor to a sitting position.

4. Transitions from standing to floor and vice versa should be performed carefully.

5. Modifications for low-impact aerobics:

    a. The traditional large, low, down-up step patterns performed in low-impact aerobics can cause pelvic floor pressure, knee stress and compromised balance. Modify these movements by reducing down-up motion and incorporating more traveling movements instead.

    b. Upper-body motion should include both long- and short-range movements to avoid excessive stress on the shoulder joints.

V. Overview of Exercise for the Pregnant Woman

A. Goals

1. Pregnancy is not the time to make large gains in fitness levels. The goal of an exercise program prescribed in conjunction with pregnancy is to maintain the highest level of fitness consistent with the individual's pre-pregnancy fitness level, and the maximum safety for both mother and child.

2. Pregnancy is usually the most physiologically stressful period of a woman's life. A safe and effective fitness program performed before, during and after pregnancy can help in the body's adjustment to the various stages and may help prevent permanent problems such as lower back strain or weakened pelvic floor muscles.

3. Weight loss should not be a desired goal during pregnancy. However, exercise may be useful as part of a complete prenatal program in preventing excessive weight gain.

B. Expectations

1. Exercise during pregnancy does not guarantee any of the following:

    a. a pregnancy free from discomfort or obstetrical complications

    b. a shorter, easier labor .

    c. an uncomplicated delivery with reduced incidence of cesarean section.

    d. a healthier baby.

2. Realistic expectations that are consistent with the goals outlined above should be discussed with each student.

C. Role of the Instructor

1. For both physiological and psychological reasons, attending an exercise class may be a stressful experience for a pregnant exerciser. The instructor should be cognizant of this and should try, through reassurance, education and communication with the student's physician, to alleviate as much stress as possible.

2. Specific positive skills, which an instructor should develop for teaching pregnant exercisers, include:

    a. maintaining a professional attitude that encompasses an unprejudiced and nonjudgmental attitude toward the participants.

    b. demonstrating sincere interest in developing a rapport with each participant.

    c. recognizing individual differences in fitness and health levels.

    d. adapting exercise programs to meet individual needs.

    e. being sensitive to the participants' goals and helping them establish realistic goals.

    f. identifying class participants who need more support or more personalized attention.

    g. showing sensitivity, patience and personal interest in each woman and her pregnancy.

    h. remembering the body sensitivity of pregnant women and encouraging conservative fitness attire.

    i. respecting your own area of expertise and that of other professionals by making referrals at all times when questions arise outside your professional experience and education.

VI. Pre-Class Instruction

A. See "Basic Exercise Standards and Guidelines," section IV.

B. Reemphasize

1. The importance of consistent physician-directed prenatal care.

2. The Exercise Danger Signs outlined in section III.G of this chapter.

C. Special Clothing Requirements

1. All participants should wear lightweight, non-restrictive clothing. Some participants may be more comfortable in stretch pants and T-shirts than in tights and leotards.

2. Support tights designed for pregnancy may aid in improving circulation to the lower legs.

3. Each participant should wear a supportive bra.

4. Vinyl clothing that retains body heat should not be allowed.

5. Proper shoes with a good arch support are highly recommended.

D. Review of Special Exercise Considerations

1. Review the special exercise considerations outlined in section III of this chapter with all new students.

VII. Warm-Up

A. Purpose

See "Basic Exercise Standards and Guidelines," section V.A.

B. Time

8 to 12 minutes of a balanced combination of static stretches and smoothly performed rhythmic limbering exercises.

C. Method

See "Basic Exercise Standards and Guidelines," section V.C-H.

D. Special Considerations

1. Due to increased weight and displaced center of gravity, rhythmic movements should follow a more gradual build-up and start out very basic. A fast warm-up with a lot of arm movements above shoulder height may elevate the student's heart rate too quickly. Students are less likely to lose balance or alignment if warm-up is performed on the floor. Warm-up performed on the floor allows greater stability for back and knees.

2. Warm-ups for the lower leg and foot should be included. This will increase circulation to the lower extremities and perhaps decrease edema.

3. Warm-up movements and stretches for the hip flexors and lower back should also be performed.

4. Avoid prolonged motionless standing, as this can decrease cardiac output, i.e. keep the legs moving while performing upper-body stretches or rhythmic limbering exercises.

E. Precautions

1. Unsupported forward spinal flexion can be extremely hazardous to the lumbar spine due to the extreme downward gravitational pull of the added weight of the uterus.

2. Students should be cautioned against movements that require excessive bouncing or jarring. See section III.I.1c of this chapter.

VIII. Aerobics

A. Purpose

See "Basic Exercise Standards and Guidelines," section VI.

B. Time

Cardiovascular training during class should not exceed 20 to 30 minutes for the less fit pregnant student, including pre-aerobic warm-up up to post-aerobic cool-down (see section III.A-B of this chapter).

C. Method

1. Low-impact aerobics (one foot remains in contact with the floor at all times) is the recommended method for attaining cardiovascular conditioning in a group exercise setting.

2. Start slowly and gradually increase the intensity and range of motion of the movements. Movements should be controlled and non-ballistic.

D. Special Considerations

1. Heart rate should be maintained within 55% to 70% of estimated maximum heart rate (75% for the more fit pregnant exerciser), not exceeding 144 bpm. Remember, these are generalized guidelines which may not be appropriate for every individual.

2. See section III.A.1 of this chapter for specific exercise intensity guidelines.

3. See section IV.B of this chapter for specific movement guidelines.

E. Additional Precautions

1. Novice exercisers often have difficulty pacing themselves. Be alert for signs of overexertion.

2. Heart rate should be monitored every 4 to 5 minutes during cardiovascular conditioning.

F. Alternate Aerobic Exercise

1. High-impact activities, such as running or high-impact aerobics, may be appropriate to continue during pregnancy if the individual has participated in these activities for at least 6 months prior to becoming pregnant. These individuals may have sufficient muscular development to provide joint stability for high-impact programs.

2. Pregnant exercisers who have been doing step aerobics for up to 6 months prior to pregnancy may continue as long as they have their physicians' approval. AFAA strongly recommends that step height not exceed 6 inches and be reduced to 4 inches or just the platform during the last trimester. In addition, choreography should be kept simple, with no rapid twisting movements, rapid directional changes or

propulsion movements. Straddling the bench may also become difficult as pregnancy progresses. AFAA does not recommend starting a step aerobics class during pregnancy due to the coordination and balance required to adapt to this form of movement.

3. Alternative exercises requiring low to non-impact are walking, swimming and stationary cycling. These methods may be suitable for most individuals as weight-bearing stress is limited. The maternal adaptations to both the physiological and anatomical changes appear to favor non-weight-bearing exercise over weight-bearing exercise.

4. Always require students to consult their physician prior to making any changes in their approved fitness program.

IX. Post-Aerobic Cool-Down

A. Purpose, Time and Method

See "Basic Exercise Standards and Guidelines," section VII.A-D.

B. Heart Rate

Recovery heart rate should be below 60% of estimated maximum heart rate prior to proceeding with additional exercises. Recovery heart rate (how quickly one attains pre-exercise rate) is a good indicator of whether or not the individual was exercising at appropriate intensity.

1. The post-aerobic cool-down heart rate may become more variable in the last trimester.

2. If students are only training at 60% of estimated maximum heart rate, recovery heart rate should be significantly lower to indicate adequate recovery.

C. Special Considerations

This is a very good time for students to visit the restroom and take a drink of cool water (approximately 8 oz.).

X. Upper Body Exercises

A. Purpose

To strengthen the muscles of the arms, chest, shoulders and upper back. Strengthening of these muscles could help prevent kyphosis and other postural deviations. Added weight of the breasts and the stress of carrying an infant in arms renders strengthening of the upper body extremely important if muscular strain is to be avoided.

B. Time

5 to 7 minutes

C. **Method**

   See "Basic Exercise Standards and Guidelines," section VIII.A-E.

D. **Special Considerations**

   1. See section III.E.2 of this chapter for discussion of kyphosis and its relationship to muscular strengthening.

   2. Movements should be resistive, smooth, controlled and slow enough to allow for complete extension.

E. **Push-ups**

   See "Basic Exercise Standards and Guidelines," section VIII.F.

   1. After the first trimester, push-ups should only be performed in a standing position against a wall. Traditional push-ups on the floor may be hazardous for the following reasons:

      a. Gravitational pull of added weight of uterus pulling against lower back.

      b. Placing body weight on writs aggravates risk of carpal tunnel syndrome.

F. **Precautions**

   1. Avoid jerky or rapid movements which may stress the elbow and shoulder joints.

   2. Consider keeping the legs moving with simple movements in order to avoid prolonged periods of standing.

   3. Weights of 1 to 3 pounds may be considered during pregnancy provided the student can maintain proper form and execution throughout entire workout. Heavier weights, especially if the use of weights was an established part of the student's pre-pregnancy exercise program, may be used with a physician's approval. The use of rubber bands or tubing may exacerbate carpal tunnel syndrome due to students "breaking" the alignment of their wrists with the forearm. A physician's approval is recommended for the use of any type of weights or other resistive equipment during pregnancy.

   4. Holding one's breath should be avoided. See section III.F of this chapter for specific breathing guidelines.

XI. Standing Pelvic Tilt

A. **Purpose**

   1. Teach correct body alignment.

   2. Provide strengthening potential for abdominals, buttocks and pelvic floor muscles.

   3. Stretch muscles of the lumbar spine.

B. Time

1 to 2 minutes

C. Alignment

Stand with knees aligned over toes and lower end of pelvis tilted slightly forward. See "Basic Exercise Standards and Guidelines," section I.E.

D. Method

1. Slowly release pelvis.

2. Slowly return pelvis to starting position by contracting abdominals and buttocks.

3. Pelvic floor muscles should also be contracted.

E. Precautions

1. Do not bear down on pelvic floor as this could contribute to vaginal varicosities.

2. Perform this exercise in a slow, controlled manner. Throwing the pelvis back and rapidly arching the back may strain the lumbar spine.

XII. Legs, Hips and Buttocks Exercises

A. Hips, Outer Thighs and Inner Thighs

1. Purpose

   To strengthen the muscles of the inner and outer thigh. Strengthening of adductor muscles is important when pushing during delivery. Strengthening of the gluteus medius, gluteus minimus and tensor fascia latae is important for support of the pelvic joints.

2. Time

   8 to 10 minutes

3. Alignment

   See "Basic Exercise Standards and Guidelines," section IX.C-F.

4. Special Considerations

   a. Side-lying position
      i. Abduction above 45 degrees or shoulder height in this position may strain both the lower back and/or the round ligaments.

ii. In this position, adduction exercises which require the upper leg to cross over the working leg may be difficult because of uterus size. Resting upper leg on 1 to 2 pillows will reduce stress on the pelvis and maintain better alignment.

iii. In this position, it is recommended that the head rest on the extended arm. Supporting the upper body on elbows or wrists may cause stress to the shoulders or wrists.

b. All-fours position

i. This position, often used for both abduction and to work the gluteus maximus, may be difficult during pregnancy.

1) Enlarged uterus causes increased pull on lower back and hips.

2) Supporting body weight on wrists may aggravate carpal tunnel syndrome.

3) Enlarged uterus may cause pressure on diaphragm.

4) Maintaining proper hip alignment while abducting leg is more difficult during pregnancy.

ii. The all-fours position is not recommended during the third trimester and should be used with caution for women in their second trimester.

c. Supine position

i. This position, often used for hip adduction exercises, is not recommended in the third trimester. In an unsupervised, home exercise program, the American College of Obstetricians and Gynecologists recommends no exercises be performed in the supine position after the fourth month of gestation is completed.

1) Time in supine position is limited—5 minutes or less. (see section III.I,4 of this chapter).

2) Size of enlarged uterus makes movement of legs toward midline difficult.

3) Tendency toward lordosis increases difficulty of keeping the lower back on the floor.

ii. An alternative position would be to place a pillow or two under the head and shoulders, keeping the head higher than the abdomen in order to reduce vena cava compression. Place both feet on the floor no greater than hip width apart, knees bent. While maintaining a pelvic tilt, open knees and contract adductors as you bring knees together.

B. Buttocks and Hamstrings

1. Purpose

To strengthen the gluteal and hamstring muscles which will assist in maintenance of pelvic tilt.

2. Time

4 to 6 minutes

3. Positions and Methods

See "Basic Exercise Standards and Guidelines," section IX.G, I and L.

a. Side-lying or supine

    i. Alternately contract and release gluteal muscles.

    ii. In supine position, no more than 5 minutes should be sustained (see section III.I,4 of this chapter).

    iii. The supine position may be performed prior to the fourth month.

b. All-fours position

    i. Observe considerations listed above for exercises performed on all fours (see section XII.A,4b of this chapter).

    ii. With leg bent at knee, perform thigh lifts, pushing heel toward ceiling while gluteus muscles contract.

    iii. To work one leg behind body at hip level, bend or curl lower leg, bringing heel toward buttocks. Extend and repeat. If hip flexors are tight or student suffers from round ligament syndrome, full extension of the leg behind the body to hip height may be difficult.

c. Standing

    i. Students may use a ballet barre or wall for balance.

    ii. Gluteal muscles are worked as described above by pushing heel away from body, keeping knee bent and buttocks contracted.

    iii. Hamstring muscles are worked as described above by curling the working leg in toward the buttocks, and then extending.

4. Precautions

a. Exercises on all fours or in a standing position may strain hip flexors, round ligaments and/or lower back.

    i. Hip flexor strain is more likely if long lever (straight leg) movements are performed, versus short lever (bent knee).

    ii. Strain is more likely in third trimester.

b. Due to increasing lordosis, proper alignment becomes more difficult as pregnancy progresses.

C. Quadriceps

1. Purpose

To strengthen the quadriceps muscles so that muscles in the front of the leg will assist in lifting activities reducing strain on the lower back. If student can execute pliés or lunges correctly without support, these exercises will aid in developing balance and adjusting to changing center of gravity.

2. Time

   3 to 4 minutes

3. Alignment for standing position

   See "Basic Exercise Standards and Guidelines," section IX.J.

   a. Pelvic tilt should be maintained.

   b. Knees should be aligned over toes.

4. Method

   Maintaining proper alignment, perform smaller knee bends at a moderate speed. Encourage students to contract their pelvic floor muscles as they bend their knees.

5. Special Considerations

   a. Due to instability caused by displaced center of gravity, lunges performed by stepping forward with knee bent, then stepping back, should be avoided after the first trimester. This type of lunge may stress knee ligaments. Lunges in a stationary position are appropriate if executed correctly.

   b. Deep knee bends should be avoided due to potential stress to knee ligaments.

   c. The traditional weight lifters squat may be too stressful after the first trimester due to difficulty of maintaining correct torso alignment.

6. Alignment and method for sitting or supine position

   See "Basic Exercise Standards and Guidelines," section IX.K.

   a. For limitations in a supine position, see section III.I,4 of this chapter.

   b. As alternative to the supine position, place a pillow behind the lower back, and use the hands to support the upper body. Create a semi-reclining position with pelvic tilt maintained.

7. Special Consideration

   a. Due to increased lordosis, students should be carefully monitored to make sure lower back remains on floor at all times.

XIII. Lower Back Exercises

A. Torso Stabilization

The ability to contract and stabilize with the abdominal muscles to effectively perform lower back strengthening exercises (using the erector spinae as a primary mover for spinal extension) is difficult during pregnancy. However, indirect strengthening through torso stabilization exercises is considered appropriate during pregnancy, provided students can execute the exercises correctly. See "Basic Exercise Standards and Guidelines," section VIII.G.

XIV. Abdominal Exercises

A. Purpose

To strengthen abdominal muscles and help provide support for the internal organs and the back.

B. Time

3 to 4 minutes

C. Alignment and Method

See "Basic Exercise Standards and Guidelines," section XI.C-1.

D. Special Considerations

1. Diastisis Recti

   a. Hormones soften central seam of recti muscles (linea alba).

   b. Abdominal muscles and seam stretch to accommodate growing baby.

   c. Weight of uterus falls on front of abdominal wall.

   d. Separation of recti muscles frequently occurs during pregnancy.

      i. Separation is painless except for possible chronic backache.

      ii. If separation has occurred, a gap or bulge in central abdominal area will appear while performing abdominal curl-up.

      iii. If separation has occurred, abdominal curls should be performed with splinting (place hands across separation, holding muscles together during contraction of recti muscles.

      iv. Avoid oblique work if separation has occurred.

      v. Avoid curl-ups entirely if separation measures more than 3 fingers in width.

         1) See section XIV.F, 2b-c of this chapter for alternate exercises.

   e. Supine Hypotensive Syndrome

      i. Individuals with this condition should not exercise in a supine position.

2. Perform abdominal curls slowly.

   a. Avoid fast oblique exercises that may strain round ligaments.

   b. Perform curls at half-time tempo of music.

3. Position and movement considerations

   a. As the uterus enlarges, the degree to which the head, neck and shoulders are lifted will decrease.

    b. Performing curls with feet elevated becomes increasingly difficult and should be avoided by the third trimester.

F. Precautions

1. Because of the pressure of the enlarged uterus on the vena cava in the supine position (see section III.I,4 of this chapter), allow no more than 5 minutes lying on the back at a given time.

2. If student becomes symptomatic, have her roll to her left side.

    a. Use pillows to support curl-ups and oblique curls with 1 to 2 pillows behind head and shoulders so the head and shoulders are higher than the abdomen.

    b. Pelvic tilts should concentrate on using the abdominal muscles instead of the buttocks to tilt the pelvis in all-fours position. If the all-fours position is not feasible, side-lying and standing positions may be used (see section XI of this chapter). May be done in a supine position as an alternative to curl-ups in the case of a 3-finger-width separation of rectus muscle.

    c. Concentrated inward contraction of abdominal muscles while exhaling in the all-fours position, side-lying and standing positions is also appropriate. May be done in a supine position as an alternative to curl- ups in the case of a 3-finger separation of rectus muscle.

XV. Pelvic Floor Exercises

A. Purpose

To strengthen the muscles located between legs attached to pubic bone and coccyx. Important because these muscles support pelvic organs. Weak pelvic floor muscles may lead to:

1. Urinary incontinence

2. Postnatal sexual dysfunction

3. Postnatal uterine prolapse

B. Time

1 to 2 minutes in class. Should also be performed frequently throughout the day.

C. Position

Standing, sitting or side-lying-may be performed in most any position.

D. Method

Contract the muscles that a woman uses to stop the flow of urine; hold for 5 seconds, building up to 10 seconds. Release and repeat.

1. No more than 5 to 10 repetitions should be done at a given time, but students should be encouraged to perform 50 to 100 repetitions throughout the day.

2. Students should be encouraged to completely relax the pelvic floor muscle between repetitions in order to learn how to release this muscle group during pushing.

3. At the end of the repetitions, the pelvic floor muscles should be contracted slightly, not left in a relaxed state, in order to adequately support the pelvic organs.

E. **Preparation for Pushing**

1. Learning the coordination of the muscle groups used during pushing is important. Simultaneously combine pelvic tilt with relaxation of the pelvic floor muscles and inward abdominal contraction.

2. The above 3-in-1 exercise should be incorporated into classes if possible, or at least taught to the student to practice at home.

XVI. Exercising with Weights

Weights of 1 to 3 pounds may be considered during pregnancy, provided the student can maintain proper form and execution throughout the entire workout and has the consent of their physician. If the use of weights was an established part of the student's pre-pregnancy exercise program, heavier weights, especially for the quadriceps and buttocks/hamstrings, may be used with a physician's approval. However, due to potential stress on the already stressed pelvic joints, weighted workouts for the abductors and adductors should be approached with extreme caution, and are not recommended for the student who has never used resistive equipment.

XVI. Cool-Down Stretches and Final Heart Rate

A. **Purpose**

To stretch muscles involved in strengthening exercises and those muscles continually flexed because of increased and changed distribution of body weight, i.e., lower back. It is also important to determine that heart rate is within normal non-exercise range.

B. **Time**

3 to 7 minutes at the end of class

C. **Method**

See "Basic Exercise Standards and Guidelines," sections XII-XIII.

1. Only static stretches should be performed.

2. Avoid stretching to maximum muscle length.

D. Special Considerations

1. Include the "angry cat" stretch, performed on all fours, in order to stretch back.

2. Stretching on floor allows for greatest stability and balance.

3. Include stretches for the hip flexors also.

E. Precautions

1. Observe guidelines regarding standing forward flexion (see section VII.E,1 of this chapter). Forward flexion in a sitting position will become increasingly difficult as the uterus expands.

2. If lying on back, observe guidelines for supine exercise (see section III.I,4 of this chapter).

F. Final Heart Rate

1. Heart rate should be below 60% of estimated maximum heart rate.

2. Heart rate elevated above 60% of estimated maximum heart rate may indicate that student was exercising at too high of an intensity.

3. If heart rate remains elevated 5 minutes after vigorous exercise, the student's physician should be consulted.

XVII. Deep Relaxation Exercises

A. Purpose

To establish a conditioned response to control the discomfort of labor and establish a physical awareness of how to relax specific muscles.

B. Time

5 minutes; may also be practiced by students at home each evening before bed.

C. Method

Students are instructed to alternately contract and release specific muscles. Exercises vary to include muscle groups in different combinations and order of relaxation. For example:

1. Contract the muscles in both legs. Starting with the right leg, gradually release all the tension in the toes, ankle, calf, knee, and on up the leg, through the thigh to the hip. Contraction of muscles in the left leg should be maintained, thus teaching students how to isolate specific muscles.

2. Deep slow breathing should accompany relaxation.

3. Vary contraction/relaxation exercises to teach awareness of tension in the major muscle groups of the upper and lower body allowing individuals to feel the difference between a relaxed muscle and a tensed muscle.

4. Verbally instruct use of imagery to help in the relaxation process. Ask students to imagine their bodies being supported by a cloud, or all of their joints being made of Jell-O.

5. Always use a soft, near monotone voice when instructing relaxation. It may be useful to dim the lights. Soothing "mood" music, such as the sound of waves or wind will help relaxation.

References

American College of Obstetricians and Gynecologists (February, 1994). Exercise during pregnancy and the postpartum period. *ACOG Technical Bulletin*, 189.

American College of Obstetricians and Gynecologists (1985). Exercise during pregnancy and the postnatal period. *ACOG Home Exercise Programs*. Washington, D.C.

American College of Sports Medicine (1991). *Guidelines for graded exercise testing and prescriptions*. Philadelphia: Lea and Febiger.

Artal, R., Rutherford, S., Romen, Y., Kammula, R.K., Dorey, F.H., & Wiswell, R.A. (1986). Fetal heart rate responses to maternal exercise. *American Journal of Obstetrics and Gynecology*, 155.

Artal, R., & Wiswell, R.A. (1986). *Exercise and pregnancy*. Los Angeles: Williams & Wilkins.

Artal, R., & Subak-Sharpe, G.J. (1992). *Pregnancy and exericse*. New York: Delacorte Press.

Artal, R., Freeman, M., & McNitt-Gray, J. (1990). Orthopedic problems in pregnancy. *The Physician and Sports Medicine*, 18:9.

Bonds, D.R., & Delivoria-Papadopoulos, M. (1985). Exercise during pregnancy—Potential fetal and placenta metabolic effects. *Annals of Clinical and Laboratory Science*, 15.

Cassidy-Brin, G., Hornstein, F., & Downer, C. (1984). *Woman-centered pregnancy and birth*. Pittsburgh: Cleis Press.

Clapp, J.F. (1985). Fetal heart rate response to runing in midpregnancy and late pregnancy. *American Journal of Obstetrics and Gynecology*, 153.

Clapp, J.F., & Dickstein, S. (1985). Endurance exercise and pregnancy outcome. *Medicine and Science in Sports and Exercise*, 16.

Collings, C.A., & Curet, L.B. (1985). Fetal heart rate response to maternal exercise. *American Journal of Obstetrics and Gynecology*, 151.

Collings, C.A., Curet, L.B., & Mullinax, J.P. (1983). Maternal and fetal responses to a maternal aerobic exercise program. *American Journal of Obstetrics and Gynecology*, 145.

Cummings, S. (January, 1986). The pregnant pause. *Health Magazine*.

Dressendorfer, R.H., & Goodlin, R.C. (1986). Fetal heart rate response to maternal exercise testing. *The Physician and Sports Medicine*, 14.

Gauthier, M.M. (1986). Guidelines for exercise during pregnancy: Too little or too much. *The Physician and Sports Medicine*, 14.

Goodlin, R.C., & Buckley, K.K. (1984). Maternal exercise. *Clinics in Sports Medicine*, 3.

Gorski, J. (1985). Exercise during pregnancy: Maternal and fetal responses. *Medicine and Science in Sports and Exercise*, 17.

Hall, D.C., & Kaufman, D.A. (1987). Effects of aerobic and strength conditioning on pregnancy outcomes. *American Journal of Obstetrics and Gynecology*, 157.

Holstein, B.B. (1988). *Shaping up for a healthy pregnancy*. Champaign, Ill.: Life Enhancement Publications.

Hutchinson, P.L., Cureton, K.J., & Sparling, P.B. (1981). Metabolic and circulatory responses to running during pregnancy. *The Physician and Sports Medicine*, 9.

Jones, B.R., Botti, J.J., Anderson, W.M., & Bennet, N.L. (1985). Thermoregulation during aerobic exercise in pregnancy. *Obstetrics and Gynecology*, 65.

Kattus, A.A. (1972). Exercise testing and training of apparently healthy individuals: A handbook for physicians. New York: American Heart Association Committee on Exercise.

Ketter, H.G., & Emerson, K., Jr. (1984). Pregnant and physically fit too. *American Journal of Maternal Child Nursing*, 9.

Kulpa, P.J., White, B.M., & Visscher, R. (1987). Aerobic exercise in pregnancy. *American Journal of Obstetrics and Gynecology*, 156.

Lokey, E., Tram, Z.V., Wells, C., Myers, B., & Tran, A. (1991). Effects of physical exercise on pregnancy outcomes: A meta-analytic review. *Medicine and Science in Sports and Exercise*, 23.

Lotgering, F.K., Gilbert, R.D., & Longo, L.D. (1985). Maternal and fetal responses to exercise during pregnancy. *Physiological Reviews*, 65.

Metcalfe, J., McAnulty, J.H., & Ueland, K. (1981). Cardiovascular physiology. *Clinical Obstetrics and Gynecology*, 24.

Nagy, L., & King, J. (1983). Energy expenditure of pregnant women at rest or walking self-paced. *American Journal of Clinical Nutrition*, 38.

Nilsson, L.A. (1986). *A child is born*. New York: Dell.

Noble, E. (1988). *Essential exercises for the childbearing year*. Boston: Houghton Mifflin Co.

Pernoll, M.L., Metcalfe, J., & Paul, M. (1978). Fetal cardiac response to maternal exercise. In L.D. Longo & D.D. Reneau (Eds.), *Fetal and Newborn Cardiovascular physiology*, 2.

Platt, L.D., Artal, R., Semel, J., Sipos, L., & Kammula, R.K. (1983). Exercise in pregnancy II: Fetal responses. *American Journal of Obstetrics and Gynecology*, 147.

Pleet, H., Graham, J., & Harvey, M. (1980). Patterns of malformaitons fesulting from teratogenic effects of trimester hyperthermia. *Pediatrics*, 14.

Pomerance, J.J., Gluck, L., & Lynch, V.A. (1974). Physical fitness in pregnancy: Its effects on pregnancy outcome. *American Journal of Obstetrics and Gynecology*, 119.

Rote, B., & Sekine, K. (1987). The educational needs of the prenatal patient who participates in dance exercise. *Topics in Acute Care and Trauma Rehabilitation*, 22.

Shangold, M., & Mirkin, G. (1985). *The complete sports medicine book for women*. New York: Simon and Schuster.

Sibley, L., Rhuling, R.O., Cameron-Foster, J., Christensen, C., & Bolen, T. (1981). Swimming and physical fitness during pregnancy. *Journal of Nursing-Midwifery*, 26.

Ueland, K., Novy, M.J., Peterson, E.N., & Metcalfe, J. (1969). Maternal cardiovascular dynamics IV: The influence of gestational age on the maternal cardiovascular response to posture and exercise. *American Journal of Obstetrics and Gynecology, 104.*

Veille, J.C., Hohimer, A.R., Burry, K., & Speroff, L. (1986). The effects of exercise on uterine activity in the last eight weeks of pregnancy. *American Journal of Obstetrics and Gynecology, 155.*

Wallace, A.M., Boyer, D.B., Dan, A., & Holm, K. (1986). Aerobic exercise and maternal self-esteem and physical discomforts during pregnancy. *Journal of Nursing-Midwifery, 31.*

Wallace, A.M., & Engstrom, J.L. (1987). The effects fo aerobic exercise on the pregnant woman, fetus and pregnancy outcome: A review. *Journal of Nursing-Midwifery, 32.*

Wells, C.L. (1985). *Women, sports and performance.* Champaign, Ill.: Human Kinetics.

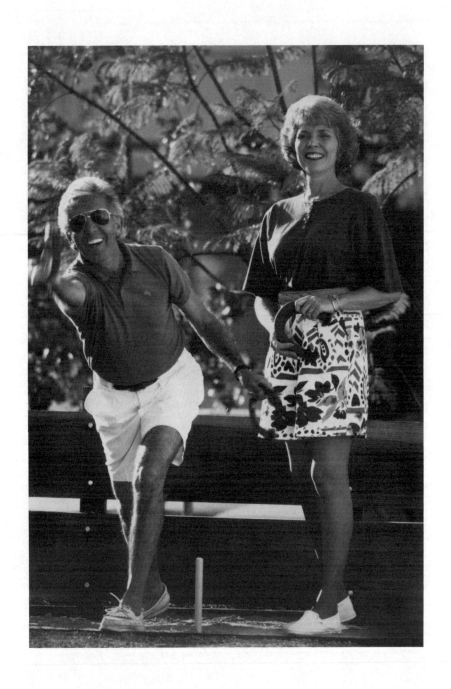

STANDARDS AND GUIDELINES

of the

Aerobics and Fitness Association of America

for

Senior Fitness

Part I: Healthy Sedentary Mature Adults

Preface:

Regular physical activity has been demonstrated to be a positive measure in helping the elderly carry out general daily tasks. Experts have shown that exercise is a must, no matter what age we are, and maintaining a regular exercise program throughout our lives may lead to a more rewarding life. The primary goal of any exercise program should be to improve or maintain health. Aside from the health benefits, consistent, progressive exercise has also been shown to be one of the key factors in successful aging.

Many instructors have lacked the knowledge and confidence to provide safe and effective fitness programs for seniors. Due to society's stigma on aging and the elderly's fear of exercise, very few programs have been developed for this special population which suffers from heart disease, diabetes, arthritis, osteoporosis, etc. With more research being conducted and a greater confidence level established within the medical profession concerning exercise prescription for the elderly, our society is beginning to see a rise in the need for the development of physical fitness programs for seniors as well as qualified instructors to teach them.

For health care and fitness professionals who are interested in senior fitness, the following questions may be of concern: how much exercise is too much and what types of exercise are contraindicated? AFAA, through the research of many respected individuals in the fields of gerontology, exercise physiology and fitness instruction, now proposes these standards and guidelines for safe and effective exercise for the average healthy, ambulatory senior participant. These guidelines are designed to be used in conjunction with the "Basic Exercise Standards and Guidelines of the Aerobics and Fitness Association of America" in AFAA's *Exercise Standards & Guidelines Reference Manual*. Guidelines for the disabled, nonambulatory and/or institutionalized elderly are addressed in "Part II: Therapeutic Exercise Programming for the Frail, Disabled, Nonambulatory and/or Institutionalized Elderly." Since seniors come in all shapes and sizes as well as all fitness levels, please also refer to "Standards and Guidelines of the Aerobics and Fitness Association of America for the Overweight Participant" in AFAA's *Exercise Standards & Guidelines Reference Manual*.

Definitions:

Aging—refers to the regular changes that occur in mature, genetically representative organisms living under representative environmental conditions as they advance in chronological age (Birren & Renner, 1977). According to Waneen Spirduso, author of *Physical Dimensions of Aging*, aging refers to a process or group of processes occurring in living organisms that, with the passage of time, leads to a loss of adaptability, functional impairment and eventually death (1995). There are different rates of aging among individuals. For example, one may appear old yet his or her psychological and social capacities for adaptation and change may be similar to (or even more advanced than) individuals half his or her age (Ostrow, 1984). An 81-year-old man may have the ability to run longer and faster than a 60-year-old man.

Gerontology—refers to the study of the normal processes of development, the differences found among people of all ages, as well as their causes and attenuating factors.

Basic activities of daily living (BADLs)—refers to such activities as drinking from a cup, feeding from a dish, dressing, grooming, washing or bathing, and transferring (moving from one position to another).

Instrumental activities of daily living (IADLs)—refers to activities such as light house cleaning, preparing dinner, washing and ironing clothes, and shopping.

Activities of daily living (ADLs)—refers to activities such as eating and drinking, going up and down stairs, moving outdoors on flat ground, getting in and out of bed, and rising from a chair.

Advanced activities of daily living (AADLs)—refers to activities such as gardening, woodworking, basic house maintenance, and recreational activities (e.g., swimming, walking, hiking and biking).

Chronological Age Categories for the Mature Adult:

Middle Age	Ages 40–64: the pre-retirement years
Young Senior	Ages 65–74: the immediate post-retirement years when there is relatively minimal functional impairment
Old Senior	Ages 75–84: some functional impairment but most individuals can still live somewhat independently
Very Old Senior	Ages 85+: greater functional impairment and may need institutionalized care

Physical or Physiological Age Categories of the Mature Adult:

The Physically Elite are an unusual group in our society. They are individuals who compete in sporting events (such as the marathon, Ironman events and in tournaments available to their age group). Other individuals under this category work in a physically demanding occupation and/or participate in higher risk activities such as weight lifting, skiing, hang gliding, and scuba diving.

The Physically Fit are individuals who perform moderate physical work, endurance exercise and hobbies. They exercise 2-3 times per week, or on a daily basis, primarily for their health, enjoyment and well-being. They do not compete or exercise as long or as intensely as those among the physically elite.

The Physically Independent are individuals who can perform very light physical work, low level hobbies such as walking and gardening, and low physical demand exercises such as golf, social dancing and traveling. Many members of the old and oldest-old age group are in this category.

The Physically Frail are individuals who may be able to perform light housekeeping, food preparation and grocery shopping with assistance. As defined by the AMA, these individuals have multiple disease processes that limit normal functional activity. They may be homebound.

The Physically Dependent are individuals who are able to perform very little physical activity, need assistance with sitting and standing, cannot perform all of the basic acitivities of daily living such as walking, bathing and dressing, and are usually in need of home or institutional care.

I.   Benefits of Exercise for Seniors

A. Physiological Benefits of Exercise

1. Increased aerobic capacity
2. Decreased resting heart rate
3. Decreased blood pressure
4. Reduced blood serum cholesterol and triglycerides
5. Increased muscle strength and endurance
6. Increased muscle mass and neural response
7. Improved circulation
8. Reduced body fat
9. Improved sleep

B. Musculoskeletal Benefits of Exercise

1. Increased muscle strength and endurance
2. Increased bone density
3. Increased range of motion
4. Increased flexibility
5. Improved joint stability
6. Improved balance
7. Improved ease of movement

C. Psychosocial Benefits of Exercise

1. Reduced tension, anxiety and fatigue

2. Enhanced feeling of well-being

3. Improved self-image and self-esteem

4. Opportunity for shared activity with friends

5. Maintenance of independence and self-care

6. Reduction of pain

II. Participant Screening

A. Medical Clearance

All individuals beginning an exercise program should follow the guidelines for medical clearance as stated in "Basic Exercise Standards and Guidelines." Additionally, to avoid risk of injury to participants and litigative risk to instructors, attendance in your class should be limited to those with physician approval. The primary responsibility for the individual's overall health management should lie with the physician. A close alliance between the fitness instructor and the participant's physician is strongly recommended.

B. Health Risk Appraisal

It is important to evaluate an individual's fitness level prior to an exercise program for the following reasons:

1. To determine the current level of physical fitness and overall health status.

2. To objectively evaluate an individual's response to exercise.

3. To determine an appropriate workload when individualizing an exercise program.

C. Role of Instructor in Health Screening Process

Only qualified specialists (e.g., physicians with the assistance of exercise test technologists or licensed, registered or certified clinical exercise physiologists) may assess the safety of exercise and administer an exercise stress test. Individual exercise recommendations and programs may be developed by senior fitness specialists or AFAA fitness practitioners based on the information received from the physician, a comprehensive health questionnaire filled out by the participant, and from physical fitness assessments. It is again recommended that all class participants have written approval from their physician. Hopefully, the individual's physician, who has recently completed a thorough physical and health history of a prospective student, will be most qualified to identify an appropriate level of exercise and any limitations. The fitness instructor's major post-screening responsibility is to administer the participant's exercise program in regard to type of exercise, duration, intensity, frequency and rate of progression in a safe and effective way.

D. Fitness Assessments

When assessing the Physically Elite, Physically Fit and the Physically Independent, it is important to follow the ACSM guidelines for testing and physician's clearance. There is no single instrument that will be appropriate in all circumstances. The instrument selected will depend upon the physical function of the mature adult and on the purpose for which the information collected is intended to be used (i.e., developing a standard of living or developing an activity program. It may also be used by a health care provider to assist in prescibing a course of treatment). When deciding on an appropriate scale or test it is important to consider certain parameters such as validity, reliability, sensitivity, acceptability, responsiveness to change and practicality.

1. The Physically Elite and Physically Fit represent approximately 5% of those individuals over 70 years of age and are capable of being assessed using the traditional physiological fitness tests. Some examples:

   a. Submaximal cardiovascular testing (YMCA protocol for bike test; modified Balke or Naughton protocol for treadmill).

   b. Strength tests (1RM is not recommended): should reflect the goals and daily activities of mature adults.

   c. Flexibility tests: should reflect the joint flexibility in the total body, not just hip and back.

   d. Functional tests: looking at mobility which represents strength, flexibility, balance, gait and activities of daily living (ADLs).

2. The Physically Independent represent approximately 70% of the elderly population. They may be experiencing physical declines that place them at greater risk of frailty. There are very few reliable and valid tools for assessing this group.

3. The Physically Frail and Physically Dependent represent approx. 25% of the older adult population and can be assessed by using a large variety of scales and indexes which have been developed for the purpose of assessing basic ADL and IADL function. Most of these tests were developed by allied health professionals for the purpose of determining rehabilitation needs and/or types of services required.

III. Training Principles and Guidelines

The factors that need to be taken into consideration when personalizing an exercise program for individuals over 60 years of age are: size, strength, flexibility, balance and coordination, orthopedic limitations, personal goals, and current health status including the presence of risk factors. From the standpoint of compliance, the participant's time schedule and exercise preference must also be considered.

A. Intensity and Duration

Research indicates exercise training at a moderate intensity (50%-70% of heart rate reserve) for a longer duration (minimum of 20-30 minutes) will lower the risk of cardiovascular disease and improve the cardiorespiratory system in the mature adult. Training at more vigorous intensities (75%-90%) will bring optimal cardiorespiratory fitness. However, these higher intensities also increase the risk of injury to seniors. Since older adults may suffer from a wide variety of medical conditions, a more conservative approach to prescribing aerobic exercise should be taken. Intensities may range from 40%-60% of heart rate reserve and the duration may be limited to several 10-minute bouts. It may help lower risk of injury by gradually increasing duration versus intensity. The utmost caution should be taken during the exercise program since exercise itself raises the systolic blood pressure during the activity. Chair aerobics has been developed as a fun and positive alternative for seniors who are unable to stand due to a degenerative disease or rehabilitation from orthopedic surgery. The Karvonen formula and the Borg Scale of Perceived Exertion are the two recommended methods for determining and monitoring training heart rate of senior participants (see Appendices).

B. **Frequency**

An exercise frequency of at least three days per week is recommended. Exercise frequency of more than five days per week and duration in excess of 60 minutes per session seems to offer the participant little additional gain in aerobic capacity yet appears to greatly increase the incidence of orthopedic injury. Just staying active on a daily basis (e.g., gardening, cleaning house, shopping, brisk walking, etc.) helps to maintain general fitness in seniors according to the 1996 U.S. Surgeon General's Report on Physical Activity and Health.

C. **Rate of Progression**

Exercise must be of sufficient duration, intensity and frequency in order to create a training effect. This training effect will usually allow the individual to increase his/her workload somewhat each class. Instructors should be watchful of these changes with each of their students and make appropriate recommendations for increasing the workload when necessary. Each student's exercise program should be evaluated and adjusted individually. Keep in mind the senior participant may demonstrate a slower rate of progression due to the aging process.

D. **Posture and Alignment**

Instructors should be particularly aware that sedentary seniors may have alignment problems due to natural aging and osteoporosis. Therefore, senior participants should be encouraged to maintain good posture and alignment whenever possible. (Refer to "Basic Exercise Standards and Guidelines," section I.,E., *Exercise Standards & Guidelines Reference Manual*.)

E. **Speed of Movement**

1. Natural changes occurring through the aging process must be taken into consideration when developing exercises for the senior participant. Due to degeneration of joint surfaces as well as a decrease in the amount and thickness of the synovial fluid in the joint, an increase in joint stiffness and loss of flexibility occurs as we age. Muscle tissue tends to atrophy causing a decrease in size of muscle fiber and muscle strength. Reaction time slows with age. Therefore, one's ability to process a given stimuli or movement pattern will decrease as will kinesthetic

awareness and balance. Because of these changes occurring with age, all movement, including stretching, calisthenics, resistance training and cardiorespiratory conditioning, should be performed with control and slow-to-moderate speed. (Refer to "Basic Exercise Standards and Guidelines," section I.,F., *Exercise Standards & Guidelines Reference Manual.*)

2. Speed of movement has a direct impact on the intensity of the exercise. As heart rate should be carefully controlled, the speed of any movement should directly correlate to the shape, size, fitness level and exercise experience of the individual.

3. Extra time should be allowed to make the transition from the floor to a standing position or vice versa. Raising or lowering the body should be accomplished slowly and carefully to avoid dizziness and injury. A chair may be utilized for support. Some seniors may not feel comfortable going down to the floor. Alternative exercises that can be performed in a standing or seated position should be demonstrated. Proper body mechanics should be utilized when lowering down to the floor.

F. Breathing

1. Breathing should follow a consistent rhythmic pattern throughout the class to avoid an increase in blood pressure. Inspire and expire through the nose and mouth in a relaxed fashion, always exhaling on the exertion. Have seniors exhale through pursed lips to help make sure they are exhaling completely.

2. Dyspnea (shortness of breath) and hypernea (rapid breathing) can be associated with sedentary aging due to a decrease in elasticity of tissues and decline in function of the respiratory system. These conditions may not only provoke fear and anxiety, but may also be caused by emotional stress. Dyspnea and hypernea usually lessen or disappear over time as long as the participant is in good health.

3. Reminders to breathe rhythmically should be made frequently throughout the class (especially during static and resistant exercises), and heart rate should be monitored more often than usual. (Refer to "Basic Exercise Standards and Guidelines," section IV.,E., *Exercise Standards & Guidelines Reference Manual.*)

G. Danger Signs

Know the Exercise Danger Signs as outlined in "Basic Exercise Standards and Guidelines," section III. A,2b. As part of the pre-class instruction, participants should be advised to inform the instructor of any pain or discomfort they may experience during the class. When working with senior exercisers, special attention must be paid to observing outward signs of physical distress and fatigue that could possibly lead to a more dangerous situation.

H. Music

Research into the effect of music on exercise performance reveals that energy expenditure generally increases while perceived exertion generally decreases when music accompanies exercise. The results may indicate that music acts as a stimulus that takes the mind away from the physical manifestations of exercise. This may have both a positive and a negative influence on the exerciser. On the positive side, music takes the participant's mind off the exercise, thereby allowing him/her to accomplish more of the workload with less awareness of discomfort or fatigue. On the negative side, the lessened awareness may cause a participant to exercise too strenuously, making him/her more prone to injury or exceeding his/her training heart rate. The fitness instructor should be watchful of any indicators that a participant is over exercising as a result of involvement with the music.

Music selection should be enjoyable to the senior exerciser. Music may be used for background accompaniment or for choreographed routines. When using music for choreography, make sure the tempo is appropriate for the senior participant. When moving to each beat of the music, the following beats per minute (bpm) are recommended:

1. Warm-up: 80-120 bpm (the less fit the student, the slower the tempo)

2. Aerobic conditioning: 120-149 bpm

3. Major muscle strength and endurance: 118-135 bpm

Another consideration regarding music is the volume. Volume of the music should be kept at a minimum (60 decibels is considered normal). To ensure that participants are able to hear your instructions, keep the music volume low. Also, the mature adult may become more sensitive to higher volume and certain pitches of sound. Those wearing hearing aids may need to adjust them according to the volume of the music.

I. Special Exercise Considerations

Keep in mind that the average sedentary senior may initially have difficulty meeting the minimums of exercise frequency, intensity and duration. The exercise training minimums should be incorporated only at such time as the participant is physically able to accomplish them without injury, elevated heart rate or muscle fatigue. To avoid these anxiety-producing consequences of over exercise, a low-intensity interval training program may be considered as an option for certain individuals. This allows the instructor to alternate exercises which sustain a higher heart rate with those that do not. Balance a participant's fitness level with his/her willingness to commit time to an exercise program and always offer a range of frequency, duration and intensity.

The instructor should also be aware that more seniors than ever before are having hip and knee replacements. A new prosthesis allows them to participate both in routine activities of daily living and in physical exercise with minimal or no discomfort. When self-limiting pain becomes less accurate as an indicator of the extent of safe exercising, the risk of injury to the joint may increase causing loosening or dislocation of the newly implanted prosthesis. Exercise should involve only smooth, controlled movements performed cautiously and deliberately at a slow-to-moderate speed. Instructors may also want to consult with a physician regarding exercises that are appropriate for knee and hip replacement patients.

J. Hydration

Some seniors are at greater risk of dehydration due to insufficient fluid intake and the use of diuretics for the treatment of cardiovascular disease. Caffeine and diuretics increase the body's need for fluids, and diuretics can affect the electrolyte balance within the elderly. Encourage senior participants to drink plenty of water before, during and after exercise. (Refer to "Basic Exercise Standards and Guidelines," section, XIII.,E., *Exercise Standards & Guidelines Reference Manual.*)

K. Environmental Considerations

1. Exercise programs should be conducted in well-ventilated areas with mild temperatures and relatively low humidity.

2. When exercising outdoors, temperatures should range from 40-75° F with humidity less than 60%.

3. When days register high air pollution, it is preferable to exercise indoors.

4. Participants should be encouraged to dress according to the weather conditions. In the cold, dress in layers to help keep moisture away from the body and cover the head to prevent heat loss. In the heat, dress in light, non-restrictive clothing, that allows for breathability and evaporation of perspiration.

IV. Class Format

A. Sequence

Refer to "Basic Exercise Standards and Guidelines," section II., A-B., *Exercise Standards & Guidelines Reference Manual.*)

Sequence takes on greater importance with the senior exerciser as the transition from a standing position to the floor is not always easily accomplished. It may be preferable in some cases to do the complete class in a standing or seated position to avoid the strain of lifting and lowering the body off the floor. If floorwork is to be included, place it at the end of your class to allow for adequate time to recover and return to a standing position.

B. Types of Movement

1. Aerobic exercise, which utilizes the large muscle groups and is rhythmic in nature, is preferred for cardiovascular conditioning.

2. Both aerobic and anaerobic weight-bearing exercises are recommended for stimulating bone density in the senior participant. Weights should only be used during the anaerobic/strength conditioning portion and only when the participant has reached a fitness level that would enable him/her to add the extra force outside gravity alone. Refer to "AFAA's Standards and Guidelines for Weighted Workouts," section I., B-D., *Exercise Standards & Guidelines Reference Manual.*)

3. Movements which work through the full range of motion and static stretching exercises which increase flexibility are beneficial for the senior participant.

4. Physical limitations may be more prevalent in the senior participant. Physical strength in general may be a limiting factor in and of itself. Orthopedic problems in the elderly that the fitness instructor may encounter are shoulder, hip, knee, ankle, finger

and wrist discomfort associated with arthritis. Weight-bearing activities may be alternated with non-weight-bearing activities (e.g., seated chair exercises or exercises performed in water). These methods allow avoidance of undue stress on the joints, support for a frail body and added confidence necessary for the participant to successfully complete the exercise.

5. Balance is thought to be an important factor relative to the prevention of falls, which is a major concern with the elderly. Therefore, include exercises which improve body awareness and balance. A senior's fear of falling due to poor eyesight, kinesthetic awareness, balance and strength should decrease over time by incorporating strength training and supported balancing exercises with the use of a chair, a wall or a ballet barre.

V. Exercise Overview

A. For Participant

1. By attending an exercise class, the senior participant may feel a greater social and psychological accomplishment than actual physical results.

2. Senior participants are not as concerned with the competitive side of fitness as much as they are in the improved physical ease in accomplishing daily tasks and a heightened quality of life.

3. In the initial stages of training, exercises that are easily accomplished may be preferred to those that offer a challenge. Feelings of inadequacy are thereby avoided and the participant's confidence in his/her ability to succeed begins to build.

4. Senior participants may prefer exercises that are repetitive over a period of time so they are able to notice improvements in coordination, balance, strength, endurance and flexibility.

5. Not all exercises are appropriate for the senior participant as some are difficult to learn or awkward to perform. Exercise selection should be based on the instructor's knowledge of the individual abilities of the students.

6. Stretch more often than usual. This helps to alleviate stress and any discomfort in the joints as well as increases flexibility. It also can provide a pertinent break between more strenuous exercises.

B. For Instructor

1. The fitness instructor's goals for the class should coincide with those of the participants. The primary focus of the instructor should be to improve and maintain the health of the participants in a fun and safe environment.

2. The instructor should be educated in the areas of nutrition, exercise physiology, psychology and sports medicine, and understand how each relate to the aging process. They should also be well-versed in common illnesses and diseases associated with aging and how they may affect exercise programming.

3. The instructor should provide, when possible, an adequate environment for the senior exerciser.

a. An easy access to the facility

b. Bright colors to enhance visual stimulation

c. Proper lighting to avoid glare

d. Proper acoustics, including keeping stereo volume at an appropriate level

e. Proper heating and ventilation

f. Display large-print training heart rate/perceived exertion charts, large-faced clock, etc.

4. The instructor should give clear, concise instructions in every class for each exercise. Describe the exercises generically, not specifically (e.g., "Reach toward your feet" rather than "Hold onto your feet"), to accommodate the variety of strength and flexibility levels in the class.

5. The instructor should use both verbal and nonverbal cues (hand cues) for easier following. Some participants may not be able to hear the verbal cues but can see the hand cues.

VI. Role of the Instructor

A. The fitness instructor may be the one who has the greatest impact on motivating the senior participant to long-term exercise adherence. Among other things, the instructor should be able to:

1. Maintain a professional demeanor that encompasses an unprejudiced and non-judgmental attitude toward participants.

2. Act as a role model for class participants.

3. Recognize individual differences in fitness and health levels.

4. Adapt exercise programs to meet individual needs.

5. Teach proper techniques, alignment and posture.

6. Educate participants as to which exercises increase strength and endurance, reduce fat or increase flexibility. Emphasize stretching exercises for increased range of motion and flexibility, muscular strength and endurance for efficiency in performing activities of daily living, and aerobic exercise for functional fitness. All enhance the quality of life.

7. Educate participants about the positive effects exercise has on the older population, both physically and psychologically.

8. Develop the physical skills of the participants.

9. Be sensitive to the particpants' goals as well as concerns over attaining them.

10. Show sincere interest in each participant and develop a rapport that leads to a relationship based on trust.

11. Identify class participants who need more support or personalized attention.

12. Show sensitivity, compassion, patience and a good sense of humor.

13. Talk to a senior as an adult and not as a child.

14. Be able to return praise, appreciation and warmth.

15. Design the class to include social opportunities and events.

B. Instructors should hold the following credentials:

1. An undergraduate or graduate degree in a health or fitness related field (i.e., registered nurse, recreational therapist, physical therapist, physical education, exercise physiology, etc.).

2. Specific training in senior fitness programming from either organizations, associations, colleges or universities that offer such course work (e.g., AFAA's Senior Fitness Workshop and the Fitness Practitioner Certification).

3. Course work in the field of gerontology.

4. Certified in CPR and advanced first aid/emergency response.

VII. Pre-class Procedure

Refer to "Basic Exercise Standards and Guidelines," section IV. A-F., *Exercise Standards & Guidelines Reference Manual.*)

The senior participant should be advised to wear shoes appropriate to the activity as well as clothing that enables free and comfortable movement. Choice of attire should also reflect a consideration of environment and temperature/humidity.

VIII. Warm-up

Warm-up is important to the senior participant. Sudden, high-intensity exercise can result in compromised blood flow through the heart. The exercise intensity should be increased gradually.

A. Refer to "Basic Exercise Standards and Guidelines," section V, *Exercise Standards & Guidelines Reference Manual.*

B. Special Considerations

1. Older sedentary individuals may take longer to respond to the physiological changes occurring due to exercise. Therefore, 10-15 minutes for warm-up may be more appropriate to prepare the senior participant for the more vigorous activity to follow.

2. Psychological preparation should be incorporated into the warm-up by means of gradual movements and verbal motivation from the instructor.

3. Emphasis should be placed on dynamic movements that utilize the large muscle groups as well as movements that emphasize the small muscle groups found in the hands and fingers.

4. Special attention should be given to properly prepare the back and shoulders, hip, knee and ankle joints for the more vigorous exercise to follow.

5. Exercises which improve body awareness, posture and balance may be incorporated in the warm-up as well as in the cool-down. During the initial stages of exercise training, utilize support for the balancing exercises.

C. Precautions

1. Movements should be slow and controlled.

2. Dizziness may occur if the participant closes eyes, lowers head below the heart, performs twisting motion of the neck and head or rises off the floor too quickly (orthostatic hypotension—a rapid drop in blood pressure).

3. Participants with a prothesis (e.g., hip or knee replacement) should follow their doctor's exercise recommendations pertaining to joint action and range of motion.

IX. Cardiovascular Conditioning

A. Refer to "Basic Exercise Standards and Guidelines," section VI, *Exercise Standards & Guidelines Reference Manual.*

B. Special Considerations

1. Low-impact aerobics (one foot remains in contact with the floor at all times), walking, stationary cycling, swimming and a seated chair workout are the recommended methods for attaining cardiovascular/respiratory conditioning. These activities significantly lessen the amount of stress normally associated with high-impact aerobics.

2. Start slowly and gradually increase the intensity and range of motion of the movements. Movements should be controlled and non-ballistic.

3. Arm and leg elevation should directly correlate with the range of motion, flexibility and fitness level of the individual.

4. Arm and leg elevation should be varied to control heart rate and reduce the stress on the joints.

5. Combination moves requiring coordination of both arms and legs should be entered into slowly, starting with either the arms or the legs, and then adding the other.

6. Utilize only a few moves when building a combination. Keep it simple and fun.

7. Use lateral movements with caution and simplify movement patterns.

8. Repeat directions and movement patterns often.

9. Use verbal and nonverbal cues.

X. Post-aerobic Cool-down

A. Refer to "Basic Exercise Standards and Guidelines," section VII, *Exercise Standards & Guidelines Reference Manual*.

B. Special Considerations

1. Check heart rate. Recovery heart rate is a significant indicator of whether the intensity is appropriate (when available, use heart rate monitors).

XI. Arms, Chest, Shoulders and Back Strengthening

A. Refer to "Basic Exercise Standards and Guidelines," section VIII, *Exercise Standards & Guidelines Reference Manual*.

B. Special Considerations (refer to Part II., V.,E.)

1. Weakness in the upper body is common among sedentary senior participants (especially in women) due to lack of use and atrophy of muscles, and decreased neurological response.

2. Movements should be resistive, smooth, controlled and slow enough to allow for a complete contraction and extension.

3. Free weights may be used to bring about a more rapid muscular response. Free weights should only be introduced when the class participant is able to complete a non-weighted workout with resistance and at a variety of speeds. Utilization of free weights should begin with the lowest weight (one-half to one pound) with additional weight being added only at such time as the participant is able to complete the movements and designated repetitions with ease. Maximum tension and high-resistance exercises are to be discouraged for high-risk and symptomatic individuals as well as those participants with coronary artery disease (CAD).

4. The use of elastic bands and other resistive equipment may be used for upper body conditioning when not contraindicated.

5. Incorporation of push-ups should be based on the participant's strength and orthopedic limitations. Weight-supported modifications (e.g., performing push-ups against the wall from a standing position or against a chair in a seated position) may be more appropriate in the initial stages of training.

6. If strengthening exercises are to be performed outside of the class setting on strength training equipment, refer to Appendices addressing "Strength Training for Seniors."

C. Precautions

1. A weighted workout is contraindicated for the individual suffering from severe arthritis. Those with mild arthritis can achieve improved benefit through a modest resistance training program. Work closely with the individual's physician when in doubt.

2. Proper breathing techniques are extremely important for senior participants, especially those with heart disease.

3. Dynamic lifting and isometric contractions are contraindicated for the senior participant with hypertension due to the increase in systemic arterial blood pressure.

4. Muscular strength and endurance goals have been indicated as a more positive step toward improved quality of life for the senior participant.

XII. Standing Abdominal Exercise

A. Special Considerations

1. Due to the extreme difficulty of achieving a resistive muscle contraction while maintaining proper body alignment in the execution of oblique work in a standing position, it is best to perform these exercises while seated or supine. The supine and seated positions also help to alleviate any stress that may be placed on the lumbar spine and the erector spinae from uncontrolled movements.

2. When specific medical conditions do not permit a senior individual to sit or lie down in a supine position, standing abdominal work may be the only alternative. Standing abdominal contractions (e.g., pelvic tilts), when performed regularly, can help to maintain or improve the abdominal muscles within a sedentary individual.

XIII. Legs, Hip Adduction and Abduction, and Buttocks

A. Refer to "Basic Exercise Standards and Guidelines," section IX, *Exercise Standards & Guidelines Reference Manual.*

B. Special Considerations

1. It takes longer for the senior participant to physiologically respond to exercise. Therefore, start slowly with fewer repetitions, then gradually add more repetitions as the participant becomes stronger.

2. Adaptation of major muscle strengthening exercises may be performed in a standing position or seated in a chair for those individuals who may feel more comfortable and secure in either of these positions.

3. The use of light weights and other resistive equipment may be used to enhance muscular strength and endurance when not contraindicated.

4. For the frail elderly refer to "Part II: Therapeutic Exercise Programming for the Disabled, Nonambulatory and/or Institutionalized Elderly."

5. Participants with a prosthesis (e.g., hip or knee) should follow their doctor's exercise recommendations pertaining to joint action and range of motion.

XIV. Abdominal Exercises

A. Refer to "Basic Exercise Standards and Guidelines," section XI and "Standards and Guidelines for the Overweight Participant," section XV, *Exercise Standards & Guidelines Reference Manual.*

B. Special Considerations

1. Support for the head should be incorporated on an individual basis. Pillows may be brought in to help minimize stress to the cervical spine for individuals who may have developed a degree of kyphosis or upper back stiffness.

2. The use of a pelvic tilt or reverse curl for the more experienced exerciser may help alleviate any discomfort in the neck area of the senior participant.

XV. Pelvic Floor Exercises

A. Kegel Exercises

Kegel exercises work the muscles in the pelvic floor and those muscles that control urinary function. Strengthening may occur by contracting and releasing the muscles in the pelvic floor in a slow and controlled manner. These can be performed in class or at home. The participant can work these muscles by stopping the flow of urine when urinating, holding, then continuing the flow. These exercises may help to prevent or alleviate urinary incontinence in older adults.

XVI. Torso Stabilization and Back Strengthening

A. Refer to "Basic Exercise Standards and Guidelines," sections VIII.G and X, *Exercise Standards & Guidelines Reference Manual.*

B. Special Considerations

1. The prone position may be uncomfortable or cause breathing difficulties in some participants.

2. Exercises may be performed in the all-fours position as long as there are no contraindications to knees and/or wrists.

XVII. Cool-down Stretches and Final Heart Rate

Refer to "Basic Exercise Standards and Guidelines," sections XII and XIII, *Exercise Standards & Guidelines Reference Manual.*

XVIII. Deep Relaxation Exercises

A. Purpose

To establish a conditioned response to control stress and fatigue as well as to establish a physical awareness of how to relax specific muscles.

B. Time

Five to ten minutes; may also be practiced by individuals at home during the day, or evening before bed.

C. Method

Participants are instructed to alternately contract and release specific muscles. Exercises vary to include muscle groups in different combinations and order of relaxation. Examples:

1. Contract all the muscles in your face, neck and shoulders. Starting with the face, gradually release all the tension in your face, neck and shoulders. Continue on down the body, contracting and releasing each muscle group.

2. Deep slow breathing should accompany relaxation.

3. Verbally instruct the use of imagery to aid in the relaxation process (e.g., ask participant to imagine his/her body being supported by a cloud or all of the body's joints being made of Jell-O).

4. Relaxation may be enhanced by finding a quiet place, dimming the lights, using soothing music such as sounds of the wind, waves or gentle rain, and creating pleasant thoughts.

5. When verbally cueing your students, use a soft, monotone voice, speaking slowly and clearly.

STANDARDS AND GUIDELINES

of the

Aerobics and Fitness Association of America

for

Senior Fitness

Part II: Therapeutic Exercise Programming for the Frail, Disabled, Nonambulatory and/or Institutionalized Elderly

The following is a brief overview of general characteristics as well as physiological, psychoemotional and sociological differences which set the disabled, nonambulatory and/or institutionalized elderly population apart from the younger independent senior population.

- **Circumstantial and Functional Parameters:** These individuals attend an adult daycare facility, reside in a nursing home or other long- or short-term care facility, or live at home or in a private foster care setting but are dependent on the services of relative(s) or other caregiver(s). Seventy-eight percent of persons over age 85 are restricted in activity due to general weakness, declining endurance, impaired balance and gait, neuromuscular complications or recurring falls. Forty-eight percent of noninstitutionalized persons age 85 years and older require help with activities of daily life (ADL) vs. 14% ages 65-74. Functional dependency and risk of accidental injury increase with institutionalization.

- **Census:** In 1986, there were nearly 2.8 million American citizens age 85 and older. There will be approximately 5 million by the year 2000. There will be more than 7 million by 2020.

- **Application:** In working with this population, the exercise professional will normally be called upon to perform in a group setting, which offers psychosocial as well as physiological benefits to the frail elderly participant. The instructor, then must be adept at simultaneously managing a variety of medical and psychological disorders while prescribing and supervising exercise activities of the greatest general safety and benefit to the group. Therefore, the following program information is addressed primarily to the leader of group geriatric fitness classes. However, the principles utilized can also be applied by instructors who work one-on-one with individual clients.

- **Typical Group Class Profile:** Classes include members of both sexes. Age is typically at least 75 and may exceed 100 years (certain classes may include younger members with memory deficit, disorientation, Alzheimer's disease or permanent disability resulting from accidental injury). Common medical profiles may include one or more of the following: acute hearing or speech impairment, blindness, amputation, joint replacement, crippling arthritis, obesity, underweight, sensory deprivation, extreme atrophy, advanced osteoporosis, spinal injury, insulin-dependent diabetes, Parkinson's disease, multiple sclerosis (MS), cancer, stroke, chronic obstructive pulmonary disease (COPD), cardiovascular disease (CVD) and/or mental impairment.

I. Special Physiological Considerations Regarding Frail Elderly Population

A. Cardiovascular and Respiratory System

1. Changes within the cardiovascular and respiratory systems in the frail elderly population are likely to be more prevalent, to present more pronounced symptoms, and to appear at more advanced stages.

2. Additional Cardiovascular/Respiratory Concerns

   a. Peak stroke volume may decline due to a reduction of heart muscle mass, reduced myocardial contractility resulting in decreased pump force, acute varicose veins and loss in general venous tone, advanced inflexibility of the aorta combined with high systemic blood pressure, and extreme skeletal muscle weakness resulting in reduced perfusion of active limbs.

   b. Oxygen extraction may be impaired due to lowered enzyme activity, critical vessel occlusions, and a declining ratio of capillary-to-muscle fiber—all of which may, in turn, adversely affect A-VO$_2$ difference.

   c. Activities such as walking, bathing and using a bedpan may consume 80% of VO$_2$ max in frail elderly. Climbing stairs may exceed VO$_2$ max in males and females in their 80s. Autopsies performed on 90-105 year olds showed that 43% developed critical occlusive coronary artery disease.

   d. Practical aerobic exercise programming implications

      1) Conditioning can be accomplished in seated postion with sustained energetic upper body movement.

      2) Aerobic training is unlikely to reverse coronary artery disease (CAD) in this population although it may provide other benefits.

      3) Group aerobics courses: only when members have undergone graded exercise testing (GXT) (adapted as necessary); only under permanent supervision of an experienced cardiologist; only with ongoing support and monitoring (blood pressure and electrocardiogram) by qualified technical personnel; only with written medical approval.

      4) Individual aerobic training (e.g., assisted walking programs which meet aerobic frequency, intensity and duration criteria): only when instructor meets personally with client's physician to discuss medical history and

individualized exercise prescription, goals and guidelines; only with written orders of a specific nature.

5) Medical staff can decrease risk of arrhythmia by diagnosing and treating typical fluid, mineral and electrolyte imbalances.

6) This population will be subject to more extreme venous pooling than other groups after strenuous exercise. In the rare instances when criteria are met so that aerobic training can be undertaken, a long and gradual cool-down is indicated to prevent syncope (temporary loss of consciousness) and orthostasis (unable to stand).

B. Musculoskeletal System

1. Changes within musculoskeletal and body composition in the frail elderly population are likely to be more prevalent, to present more pronounced symptoms, and to appear at more advanced stages.

2. Additional Muscular Strength and Endurance Concerns

   a. In frail elderly populations, decline in lean muscle mass may affect muscular performance more dramatically. Lean mass can decline as much as 30% between ages 30 and 80. Strength declines appear to accelerate after age 75 (65% of women ages 75-84 cannot lift 10 lbs or 4.5 kg versus 45% of women ages 65-74 and 40% of women ages 55-64). Handgrip strength can be predicted to decline 21% between ages 30 and 80, while leg and back strength decline by 40%.

   b. In very old age, there is a change in character and a decline in number of satellite cells (located between sarcolemma and basal lamina of skeletal muscle fibers) which leads to a decreased, though still functioning, capacity for muscle regeneration. Therefore, although muscular injury must be avoided, muscular conditioning can safely be attempted.

   c. Practical exercise programming implications

      1) Grip strength can be improved by squeezing activity.

      2) Muscular strength and endurance gains can be successfully effected in the elderly through seated upper and lower body exercises utilizing gravity and/or low external resistance.

         a) Longer training is necessary for significant improvement (in one eight-week exercise study, 40-80 year olds all improved in muscular performance, but the gains decreased in degree with each additional decade lived).

         b) Hypertrophy is not to be expected.

3. Additional Range of Motion (ROM) Concerns

   a. In the very old, ROM deficit is often secondary to injury, chronic disease and/or enforced bed rest.

   b. Individuals in their 80s have been seen to increase flexibility to the same degree as individuals in their late teens with gentle stretch exercises.

   c. Practical exercise programming implications

1) Implement a mild, seated stretch program when not contraindicated. For example, in an 84 year old individual with ROM of both shoulder joints limited to 20-30° in all planes, improvement occurred with the following types of gentle resistive exercise: place hands behind head and rotate elbows backward; move arm within allowed ROM while holding a soup can as an added weight (approximately 10-1/2 ounces) in hand; lift broom stick with a one pound weight attached.

2) Implement a bed exercise program when necessary. For example, in a 74 year old individual incapable of sitting due to hip, knee and back contractures, successful rehabilitation occurred with cautious, conservative neck movement; rolling and reaching from side-to-side in bed; leg raises and circles; bringing knee toward chest.

4. Additional Skeletal Concerns

   a. By age 90, 1 in 3 women experience hip fractures. Practical exercise programming implications: training should address fall prevention through strengthening; gentle exercise can usually be implemented after hip surgery or replacement.

   b. In addition to other well-established risks, heavy weights (or training progression that is not gradual enough) may break down bone tissue at a faster rate than that at which the tissue can recover in frail elderly persons, leading to stress fracture.

   c. Simply standing has been seen to stimulate more bone remineralization than bicycle riding (because it is weight-bearing). In group settings, non-typical members capable of standing during upper body exercises should be encouraged to do so.

   d. When music is incorporated into classes, standing and shifting hips to the beat may also yield motivational benefits; when ambulatory Alzheimer's disease patients attend, standing may provide a positive outlet for excess, undirected energy and may be useful in the continual goal of keeping Alzheimer's disease patients satisfactorily occupied.

   e. Bone material of cervical vertebrae in frail elderly populations is subject to fracture. Contraindicated exercises: head rolls and tilting head backward—both over-compress vertebral tissue.

   f. In spinal osteoporosis, back extension exercise may help to prevent vertebral fracture, whereas back flexion may be dangerous due to over-compression.

   g. There are 26 bones in the human foot, many of which are tiny and delicate. In the very old, they may be extremely fragile and subject to fracture. In institutional settings many persons wear socks or slippers instead of sturdy shoes and many facilities have tile or terazzo floors. Practical exercise programming implications: closely supervise seated "walking," "marching" and "running" to ensure that participants touch down lightly.

C. Blood

1. Blood/Circulation Concerns

   a. In individuals malnourished due to sensory deprivation, depression or chronic disease, O_2 extraction may be paired secondary to anemia.

b. Impaired respiratory function may result in incomplete oxygenation of pulmonary capillary blood.

c. Blood flow may be redistributed, with a greater relative proportion routed to areas where O_2 extraction is limited (e.g., skin, kidneys, other viscera).

d. Practical exercise programming implications: energy level will be reduced; exercise tolerance will be reduced; aerobic capacity even for low-level stretch and calisthenic activity will be reduced; frequent and regular rest intervals are indicated (and supported by population's general tendency toward dyspnea and other signs and symptoms).

D. Metabolic and Regulatory System

1. Metabolic and Regulatory System Concerns

   a. Prevalence and incidence of incontinence increase sharply. Practical exercise programming implications: conduct classes in location with easy restroom access; assist participants to and from restroom facilities during classes if necessary; consult care plan team in order to schedule classes at times during which affected participants do not customarily have accidents.

   b. Prolonged sitting increases pressure in the abdominal region which may cause discomfort. Practical exercise programming implications: include exercises that cause a shift in weight, and bend, stretch and turn the trunk.

E. Nervous System

1. Neuromuscular Concerns

   a. Lower extremity muscle weakness combined with neural deficit has been tentatively identified as an independent risk factor for falls. Practical exercise programming implications: employ exercises that engage the knee extensors (seated leg lifts, knee lifts, knee bends, leg circles; in some cases, very light resistance might be introduced).

   b. Studies are being performed today to determine whether exercise can correct balance and gait abnormalities which lead to falls. Exercise, on the other hand does improve muscular strength in the lower extremities which reduces risk. To clarify: while a young adult uses 50% of total knee extensor strength to rise from a chair, the same activity often calls for more than 100% of an 80 year old's strength. Training can reverse this trend but will likely do so through neurological mechanisms more so than through strictly muscular mechanisms in the aged.

II. Psychosocial Considerations

A. Clincal Depression

Clinical depression has been reported in up to 20% of institutionalized elderly. Contributing factors may include loss of financial independence, personal property, privacy and control over life; feelings of helplessness, loneliness and isolation; and a tendency to withdraw.

B. Insomnia and Anxiety

Insomnia and anxiety are even more prevalent than depression among the institutionalized. Tranquilizer drugs may add to the problem by contributing to mental confusion, dependency, and drowsiness during daytime hours.

C. Practical Exercise Programming Implications

Although exercise has not been conclusively demonstrated as an effective treatment for psychosocial disorders in the oldest populations, findings regarding younger seniors can be extrapolated to support the thesis: Exercise in a group environment, when possible, is believed to be most effective by preserving social skills and by providing a sense of community and belonging.

III. Nutritional Considerations

A. In institutional settings, diet is usually supervised by a registered dietitian. However, the exercise instructor can be a more effective care team member by remembering the following:

1. Water intake should be encouraged when exercising.

2. Increased energy expenditure in institutionalized elderly (even with low-level seated stretch and calisthenic programs) may call for increased dietary intake since participants are inclined to have marginal nutrient reserves.

3. Deficiencies in zinc, potassium, magnesium and vitamin D are prevalent in this population and may interfere with motor performance. Qualified nutritional assessment is indicated in conjunction with any exercise program.

4. Commonly used drugs which can affect exercise tolerance include diuretics, insulin, beta blockers, antihypertensives and any drugs that afftect the central nervous system (CNS); medical staff should consider these implications in approving and setting guidelines for individual training.

5. Loss of appetite is a common problem among the frail elderly. Extrapolated findings obtained on younger seniors suggest exercise may be effective in stimulating appetite in the frail elderly.

IV. Exercise Goals in Frail Elderly Populations

A. Goals

1. Increase aerobic power (only under the controlled conditions stated in section I.,A.,d, of this chapter)

2. Increase muscular strength

3. Increase muscular endurance

4. Increase grip ability

5. Increase flexibility

6. Increase range of motion

7. Prevent bone demineralization and attempt remineralization

8. Decrease pressure and discomfort in abdominal region

9. Improve neurological function

10. Prevent falls and accidental injury

11. Attempt to improve gait and balance

12. Provide social contact (can be maximized through group discussion activity during rest breaks)

13. Prevent or ameliorate depression, anxiety, insomnia

14. Prevent or meliorate loss of appetite

B. Additional Goals

1. Maintenance or improvement in activities of daily life

    a. Typical activities of daily living which may be addressed: dressing, self-grooming, self-feeding, general mobility, rising from a chair or bed, and providing one's own bathroom care. Strength and stamina are also needed to engage in typical pleasurable activities such as gardening, craftwork, pet care, fishing, picnicking and attending other scheduled activities.

    b. Muscular declines limit functional activities of daily life more so than aerobic fitness declines; training should address strength, muscular endurance, flexibility and coordination.

2. Prevention of Disease

    a. Typical disorders that may theoretically be prevented in part by regular exercise include: bone loss, accidental fracture, glucose intolerance, type II diabetes mellitus and constipation.

    b. Regarding previously sedentary individuals in frail elderly populations, aerobic training is unlikely to prevent atherosclerotic disease; it may theoretically prevent or postpone cardiovascular events such as thrombosis, ischemia, angina and infarction due to positive effects on blood pressure, coagulation and lipid levels.

3. Treatment of disease (as adjunct to qualified medical attention)

    a. Exercise may contribute to overall therapy in cardiovascular disease, diabetes, stroke, Parkinson's disease, osteoporosis, arthritis, chronic obstructive pulmonary disease, chronic depression or anxiety and dementia.

    b. Exercise may improve prognosis in disease by preventing secondary complications: edema, pneumonia, pressure sores, contractures, and in some instances, pain.

V. Common Diseases of the Frail Elderly and Exercise Implications

A. Limb Amputation

1. Check stump occasionally to ensure excess rubbing of skin on wheelchair or prosthesis, which could cause irritation.

2. Position unaffected side nearer action.

B. Multiple Sclerosis, Cerebral Palsy, Polio

1. Changing from one exercise to the next may be difficult. Allow ample transition time and plenty of time with each exercise.

2. Atrophy may be considerable and ROM reduced. Select most appropriate exercises accordingly.

3. Omit all neck exercises if individual has trouble controlling head movement (rolling motions or "floppiness" increase injury risk)

C. Stroke

1. Items 1-3 under section V.B. above.

2. If paralyzed on right side, use demonstration instead of verbal instructions. Keep speech patterns short, simple and direct.

3. If paralyzed on left side, use verbal instructions instead of demonstration. Avoid quick movements or gestures.

4. Position unimpaired side closer to action.

5. Attempt to prevent neglect of impaired side by encouraging stroke patient to use stronger limb to help impaired limb complete exercise movements.

D. Diabetes

1. If insulin shot is received before exercise, injection site area should not be worked.

2. Immediately stop exercise and summon medical assistance if speech becomes slurred, if participant appears confused or bewildered or if he/she exhibits undue hunger or profuse perspiration.

3. Aged diabetics are subject to blindness and amputation secondary to circulatory disorder, and are at heightened risk of metabolic, cardiovascular and soft tissue injury with strenuous exercise. Movement must be especially gentle, conservative, pleasurable and closely supervised.

E. Arthritis

1. Encourage good standing and seated posture.

2. Due to joint damage, do not sustain any single, fixed exercise position for long periods of time.

3. Incorporate gentle, conservative ROM exercise (may include both active and passive), but never force ROM.

4. Schedule exercise during time of day when stiffness is least pronounced.

5. Arthritis may call for an exception to the general guidelines that isometric exercise should be avoided in frail elderly population. Isotonic strengthening of muscle groups at inflamed joints can aggravate tenderness and pain. In this instance, employ slow stretching and very conservative isometric work to prevent atrophy (e.g., for a short time, gently press against a wall or down on a table to engage musculature while stabilizing andprotecting affected joint). Maintain proper breathing techniques during exercise.

6. Familiarize participants with the guidelines for pain.

   a. Some aching in the muscles is to be expected and should not require altering the exercise program.

   b. Joint pain that lasts longer than one hour after exercise should be recognized as a reason to curtail a particular activity until pain subsides.

   c. Alternative or reduced activity, such as performing only range of motion exercises, is preferable to complete rest.

7. Appropriate adjustment in exercise program should be made as dictated by the overall improvement in the participant.

8. The American Rheumatism Association established criteria for classification of functional capacity.

   Class I: Complete ability to carry on all usual duties without handicaps.
   Class II: Adequate ability for normal activities despite handicaps, discomfort or limited motion at one or more joints.
   Class III: Ability limited to little or none of the duties of usual occupation or to self-care.
   Class IV: Incapacitated, largely or wholly. Bedridden or confined to a wheelchair; little or no self-care.

9. Refer to "The Other Arthritis" by Greg Welch, M.S., *American Fitness*, September/October issue, 1995.

F. Spine Injury

1. Do not stretch lower back.

2. Do not permit individual to sit in exactly the same position for more than approximately 15 minutes without shift in weight or pressure.

3. Since there are many types of spinal column injuries, consult the participant's physician for a list of exercise dos and don'ts specific to his/her particular condition.

G. Sight and Hearing Deficit

1. In order to avoid undesirable pressure or blood flow to eyes, a person with an eye-related disorder should not nod his/her head down low toward chest or lean so far forward that his/her head falls below chest level.

2. It may be helpful to guide the blind exerciser manually through movements until he/she recognizes verbal descriptions.

3. Seat hearing-impaired persons near group leader or stand besidethem when issuing instructions. Close doors leading to kitchen work areas, residence hallways and staff break rooms to minimize peripheral noise.

H. Advanced Cardiovascular Disease, Chronic Obstructive PulmonaryDisease, Inoperable Tumor, Malignancy

1. Likely to become fatigued and winded quickly.Respect self-limiting factors.

2. Encourage performance of as much medically-approved light exercise as individual feels capable of. Never prod into overexertion.

I. Osteoporosis/Osteomalacia

1. Use extremely light resistance (or if individual is quite frail, no resistance at all).

2. Pay particular attention to employing a slow, gradual progression technique.

3. Omit all spinal flexion (neck and back).Normally, back may beextended.

J. Neurologic Disease

1. Parkinson's disease is the third leading neurologic cause of disability in the aged after stroke and dementia.

   a. Participants may exhibit tremor, rigidity, speech impairment, autonomic disorder, unusual posture, shuffling gait and tendency to fall.

   b. Normally may participate in general geriatric exercise program for ROM and flexibility, muscular performance,posture improvement and coordination.

   c. Schedule exercise when rigidity is least pronounced. This will depend upon time of day medication is taken and whenpeak drug effects occur.

2. Dementia may afflict up to 30% of the very old population, age 85 plus, as compared to only 5% of all persons over 65.

   a. Individuals may exhibit disorientation as to time and place, memory loss (especially short-term), withdrawn passive behavior, aggressive disruptive behavior, inability to comprehend language and symbols (e.g., letters and numbers) and functional dependency. Alzheimer's disease may be tentatively diagnosed.

   b. A general geriatric exercise program (ROM and flexibility, muscle performance, posture, coordination) may reverse the lean tissue loss classically associated with dementia which, in turn, may prevent infections, poor wound healing, immunedeficiency and increased fraility and dependence.

   c. A general geriatric exercise program may reduce necessity for physical and chemical restraints.

   d. A general geriatric exercise program may prevent or decrease the wandering behavior and restlessness associated with Alzheimer's disease.

   e. An enclosed exercise yard may be indicated for wandering or pacing individuals.

   f. Attempt to arrest chanting or repetitive behavior with diversion techniques.

g. When possible, excuse a demented participant from group class into the care of another qualified employee if he/she cannot control disruptive behavior that is likely to upset other group members.

VI. Special Safety Considerations in Geriatric Exercise

A. Medical waiver is necessary for participants of the frail elderly in any form of individual or group exercise.

1. In facilities offering only very low-intensity seated stretching, calisthenics and short-distance gait training, the director of nursing may opt to approve participation for low-risk individuals based on a general activities waiver signed by physician.

2. Group aerobic training should not be attempted unless: all members have undergone pre-exercise screening, including graded exercise testing (GXT); the aerobics program is headed by a cardiologist; appropriate monitoring equipment and specialists are readily available to measure ongoing responses during exercise; and specific written medical orders and training methods have been issued.

3. Individual aerobic training should not be attempted unless the instructor has discussed medical history, capacity, limitations, goals and prognosis with the individual's physician and has received specific written medical approval, including individualized exercise prescription and training methods ordered.

B. Generally avoid heavy weights, isometric exercises and quick progression.

C. Keep movements smooth and gentle, and work at a slow-to-moderate rate of speed.

D. Do not remove physical restraints without medical approval.

E. Set wheelchair brakes so that chairs do not roll during seated exercises.

F. Be careful to avoid any bumping or jarring to affected areas: catheters, nasal prongs, tender spots or sores on problem feet or fingers, recent surgical and injection sites.

G. Stress Signals

1. Cease exercise and have participant rest if he/she displays or complains of lightheadedness, shortness of breath or overfatigue.

2. Cease exercise and alert medical staff at once if individual displays or complains of dizziness, severe shortness of breath, chest pain, any sharp pain, shakiness, trembling, queasiness, nausea, throbbing head, and any unusual or suspicious symptom.

3. Constantly observe students yourself for any of the signs and symptoms described above. Do not simply rely on them to communicate such responses to you.

H. Emergencies

1. Learn and practice emergency procedures followed in facility.

2. Know location of emergency call button in (or nearest to) exercise area.

3. If a situation ever develops in which you are unsure whether you should call for immediate medical assistance, do so anyway.

VII. Instructor Qualifications for Teaching the Frail Elderly

A. Refer to guidelines listed in Part I, VI.,B.

B. Additional Qualification Suggestions

1. Complete internship in applicable area(s):

   a. Cardiac/stroke rehabilitation (through local hospital clinic)

   b. Orthopedic rehabilitation (through local hospital clinic)

   c. Therapeutic recreation (can be studied by serving under a nursing home or adult day care activity coordinator)

2. Attend seminars and workshops on applicable topics:

   a. Adapted sports therapy for the elderly disabled

   b. Choreography and supervision of rehabilitative wheelchair dance

   c. Mental fitness activities programming for the elderly disabled

   d. Management and motivational techniques in geriatric exercise programming

   e. Activities management with regard to specific diseases common to the frail elderly

C. Personal Traits Needed

1. Love for the frail elderly

2. Unflagging patience

3. Good humor

4. Liveliness and warmth

5. Tact

6. Creativity

7. The ability to encourage, motivate and reward effort

VIII. Teaching Aids and Accessories

    A. Light hand weights or soup cans (from less than one lb to three-and-a third lbs)

    B. Scarves, kerchiefs—for limbering and ROM exercises

    C. Putty, clay, rubber balls, Nerf balls—for grip exercises

    D. Elastic bands (e.g.Thera-Band), Thera-Plast, surgical tubing—for muscular strengthening and endurance

    E. Music

        1. For greater flexibility and effectiveness in nursing home class management, try playing music at a low background volume solely to enhance mood and atmosphere rather than always trying to match physical movements to beat. For this purpose, music selections may include classical, gospel, big band, ragtime, show tunes, light pop, country and boogie-woogie (music may be borrowed from local libraries).

        2. Refer to Part I, III.,H.

References

Alberts, N. (April, 1995). Our aging parents: How to help. *American Health*, 54-99.

American College of Sports Medicine (1995). *ACSM's Guidelines for Exercise Testing and Prescription* (5th ed.). Baltimore, MD: Williams & Wilkins.

American College of Sports Medicine (1997). *ACSM's Exercise Management for Persons with Chronic Diseases and Disabilities*. Champaign, IL: Human Kinetics Publishers.

Anderson, T., & Kearney, J.T. (1982). Effects of three resistance programs on muscular strength and absolute and relative endurance. *Research Quarterly for Exercise and Sport*, 53(1), 1-7.

Aniansson, A., & Gustafsson, E. (1981). Physical training in elderly men with special reference to quadriceps muscle strength and morphology. *Clinical Physiology*, 1,87.

Ayalon, J., Simkin, A., Leichter, I., & Raifmann, S. (1987). Dynamic bone loading exercises for postmenopausal women: Effect on the density of the distal radius. *Archives Physical Medical Rehabilitation*, 68, 280-283.

Baylor, A.M., & Spirduso, W.W. (1988). Systemic aerobic exercise and components of reaction time in older women. *Journal of Gerontology*, 43, 121-126.

Barry, H.C., Rich, B.S., & Carlson, R.T. (1993). How exercise can benefit older patients. *The Physician and Sportsmedicine*, 22(2), 124-140.

Bell, R.D., & Laskin, J. (1985). The use of curl-up variations in the development of abdominal musculature strength and endurance by post 50 year old volunteers. *Journal of Human Movement Studies*, 11(6), 319.

Bennet, P.H. (1967). Report of work group on epidemiology. *National Committee on Diabetes*, 3(1).

Biegel, L. (1984). *Physical Fitness and the Older Person: A Guide to Exercise for Health Care Professionals*. Rockville, MD: Aspen Systems Corporation.

Birren, J.E., Wood, A.M., & Williams, M.V. (1980). Behavioral slowing with age: Causes, organization, and consequences. In L.W. Poon (Ed.), *Aging in the 1980s: Psychological Issues*. Washington, DC: American Psychological Association.

Botwinick, J. (1978). *Aging and Behavior* (2nd ed.). New York, NY: Springer.

Brooks, G.A., & Fahey, T.D. (1987). *Fundamentals of Human Performance*. New York, NY: MacMillan Publishing Company.

Brown, S.P, Cundiff, D.E., & Thompson, W.R. (1989). Implications for fitness programming-the geriatric population. *Journal of Physical Education and Dance*, 1, 18-23.

Chinnici, M. (1991). How to protect your body from time. *Self Report*, 128-129.

Clarkson, P.M., & Kroll, W. (1978). Practice effects on fractionated response time related to age and activity level. *Journal of Motor Behavior*, 10, 275-286.

Cooper Institute of Aerobic Research (1989). Senior fitness. A seminar presented at the IDEA Educational Convention, San Diego, CA.

Daleiden, S. (1990). Prevention of falling: Rehabilitative or compensatory interventions? *Topics in Geriatric Rehabilitation*, 5, 44-53.

Danner, R., & Edwards, D. (1992). Life is movement: Exercise for the older adult. *Activities, Adaptation & Aging*, 17, 15-25.

Dewitt, J., & Roberts, T. (September, 1991). Pumping up an adult fitness program. *JOPERD*, 67-71.

Dishman, R.K. (1981). Prediction of adherence to habitual physical activity. In F. Nagle & H. Montoye (Eds.), *Exercise in Health and Disease*. Springfield, IL: Charles C. Thomas.

Dishman, R.K. (1994). *Advances in Exercise Adherence*. Champaign, IL: Human Kinetics.

Duncan, P., & Studenski, S. (1992). Assessment of falls in the elderly. *Physical Therapy Practice*, 1, 69-76.

Eckert, H.M., & Espenschade, A.S. (1980). *Motor Development* (2nd ed.). Columbus, OH: Charles E. Merrill Publishing Company.

Eckert, H.M. (1987). *Motor Development* (3rd ed.). Indianapolis, IN: Benchmark Press.

Enoka, R.M. (1988). Muscle strength and its development: new perspectives. *Sports Medicine*, 6, 146-168.

Fiatarone, M.A., Marks, E.C., Ryan, N.D., Meredith, C.N., Lipsitz, L.A., & Evans, W.J. (1990). High intensity strength training in nonagenarians: effects on skeletal muscle. *Journal of American Medical Association*, 262(22), 3029-3034.

Gehlsen, G.M., & Whaley, M.H. (1990). Falls in the elderly, Part II: Balance, strength and flexibility. *Archives of Physical Medicine and Rehabilitation*, 71, 739-741.

Grabiner, M.D, & Enoka, R.M. (1995). Changes in movement capabilities with aging. *Exercise and Sport Science Reviews*, 23: 65-104.

Gryfe, C.I., Amies, A., & Ashley, M.J. (1977). A longitudinal study of falls in an elderly population: 1. Incidence and morbidity. *Age & Ageing*, 6, 201-210.

Hakim, Amy, et al., (1998). Effect of walking on mortality among nonsmoking retired men. *The New England Journal of Medicine*, 1(8): 94-99.

Johnson, C.C., & Slemenda, C. (1987). Osteoporosis: An overview. *The Physician and Sportsmedicine*, 15(11), 65-79.

Jones, D.A., Rutherford, O.M., & Parker, D.F. (1989). Physiological changes in skeletal muscle as a result of strength training. *Quarterly Journal Experience Physiology*, 74, 233-256.

Kimm, S., & Kwiterovich, P. (1995). Childhood prevention of adult chronic disease: Rationale and strategies. In L. Cheung & J. Richmond (Eds.), *Child Health, Nutrition and Physical Activity*. Champaign, IL: Human Kinetics.

La Forge, R. (April, 1995). Research: Elastic tubing and senior's strength. *IDEA Today*, 9.

Laforest, S., St-Pierre, D.M., Cyr, J., & Gayton, D. (1990). Effects of age and regular exercise on muscle strength and endurance. *European Journal of Applied Physiology*, 60, 104-111.

Larsson, L. (9182). Physical training effects on muscle morphology in sedentary males at different ages. *Medicine and Science in Sports and Exercise*, 14(3), 203-206.

Martin, J.E., & Dubbert, P.M. (1984). Behavioral management strategies for improving health and fitness. *Journal of Cardiac Rehabilitation*, 4, 200-208.

Moritani, T., & deVries, H.A. (1980). Potential for gross muscle hypertrophy in older men. *Journal of Gerontology*, 35, 672-682.

McKeag, D.B. (1992). The relationship of osteoarthritis and exercise. *Clinical Sports Medicine*, 11(2), 471-487.

Neurgarten, Havighurst, & Tobin (1961). In J.P. Robinson, P.R., Shaver, & L.S. Wrightman (Eds.), *Measures of personality and social-psychological Attitudes*. New York, NY: Academic Press (1991).

Ostrow, A.C. (1984). *Physical Activity and the Older Adult*. Princeton, NJ: Princeton Book Company.

Pyka, G., Lindenberger, E., Charette, S., & Marcus, R. (1994). Muscle strength and fiber adaptations to a year-long resistance training program in elderly men and women. *Journal of Gerontology*, 49, M22-M27.

Rikli, R.E., & Busch, S. (1986). Motor performance of women as a function of age and physical activity level. *Journal of Gerontology*, 41(5), 645-649.

Rikli, R.E., & Edwards, D.J. (1991). Effects of a three-year exercise program on motor function and cognitive speed in older women. *Research Quarterly for Exercise and Sport*, 62(1), 61-67.

Rillorta, L. (1988). Sociology of aging. Course attended at California State University, Fullerton.

Rikli, R.E., & McManis, B.G. (1990). Effects of exercise on bone mineral content in postmenopausal women. *Research Quarterly for Exercise and Sport*, 61(3), 243-249.

Roberts, S. (March/April, 1990). Active aging: Exercise and the older athlete. *American Fitness*, 51-62.

Ryff, C.D. (1989). In the eye of the beholder: Views of psychological well-being among middle-aged and older adults. *Psychology and Aging*, 4, 195-210.

Schmidt, R.A. (1982). *Motor Control and Learning*. Champaign, IL: Human Kinetics.

Serfass, R.C., et al (1985). Exercise testing for the elderly. *Topics in Gerontology Rehabilitation*, 1(1), 58.

Shephard, R.J. (1981). Cardiovascular limitations in the aged. In E.L. Smith & R.C. Serfass (Eds.), *Exercise and Aging: The Scientific Basis*. NJ: Enslow Publishers.

Shephard, R.J. (1984). Management of exercise in the elderly. *Canadian Journal of Applied Sport Science*, 9(3), 109.

Shephard, R.J. (1987). Human rights and the older worker: Changes in work capacity with age. *Medicine and Science in Sports and Exercise*, 19, 169-173.

Smith, E.L., Reddon, W., & Smith, P.E. (1981). Physical activity and calcium modalities for bone mineral increase in coed women. *Medicine and Science in Sports and Exercise*, 13, 60-64.

Spence, A.P. (1989). *Biology of Aging*. Englewood Cliffs, NJ: Prentice Hall.

Spirduso, W.W. (1980). Physical fitness and psychomotor speed: A review. *Journal of Gerontology*, 35, 850-865.

Spirduso, W.W. (1995). *Physical Dimensions of Aging*. Champaign, IL: Human Kinetics.

Stillman, R., Lohman, T., Slaughter, M., & Massey, B. (1986). Physical activity and bone mineral content in women aged 30 to 85 years. *Medicine and Science in Sports and Exercise*, 18(5), 576-580.

Tanji, J.L. (1990). Hypertension, Part I: How exercise helps. *The Physician and Sportsmedicine*, 18(7), 77-81.

Taunton, J.E., & McCargar, L. (1995). Staying active with diabetes. *The Physician and Sportsmedicine*, 23(3), 55-56.

Tinetti, M.E. (1987). Factors associated with serious injury during falls by ambulatory nursing home residents. *Journal of American Geriatric Society*, 35, 644-648.

Wankel, L.M. (1984). Decision making and social support strategies for increasing exercise involvement. *Journal of Cardiac Rehabilitation*, 4, 124-135.

Ward, A., Taylor, P., & Rippe, J. (1992). How to tailor an exercise program. *The Physician and Sports Medicine*, 19(9), 64-74.

Williams, B.R. (March, 1992). Avoiding medication misadventure. Seminar, California State University, Fullerton, Fullerton, CA.

Zadai, C.C. (1985). Pulmonary physiology of aging: The role of rehabilitation. *Topics in Gerontology Rehabilitation*, 1(1), 49.

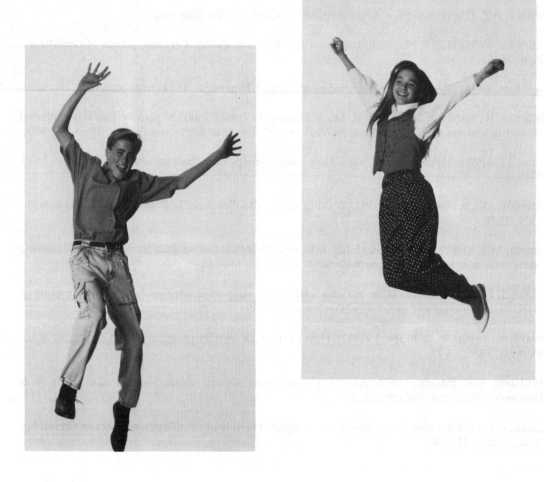
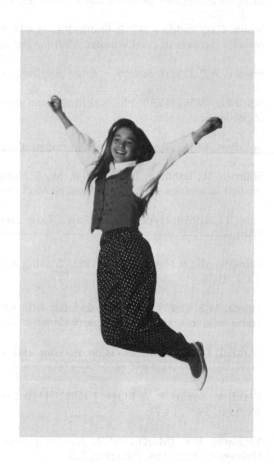

STANDARDS AND GUIDELINES

of the

Aerobics and Fitness Association of America

for

Youth Fitness Programs

Physical activity is generally considered to be an important factor in the growth and development of children and adolescents. There is a great deal of knowledge which has been generated regarding the effects of exercise on performance and health capacities in children as well as adults. And, research supports the theory that activity habits established early in life continue into adulthood. Schools have historically provided structured physical education programming for our youth. Unfortunately, many public schools nationwide are eliminating these programs from their curriculums due to financial constraints. With the decrease of activity and exercise opportunities within our schools, fitness professionals may become our primary leaders to develop youth fitness programs for their communities.

However, a need still exists to develop a general consensus on the quality and quantity of exercise required to improve and maintain a minimum level of fitness in children. The information contained in these Guidelines reflects the latest research on fitness programming for children and adolescents. Readers are encouraged, however, to keep abreast of new findings and developments in youth fitness because the field of pediatric exercise science is a relatively new and dynamic area of study. The primary focus of quality youth fitness programming is to instill an intrinsic desire for lifelong activity.

I.   Basic Principles, Definitions and Recommendations

All Standards and Guidelines apply to an average child without known physiological or medical conditions that would in any way restrict the participant's exercise activities. These Standards and Guidelines are designed to be used in conjunction with the "Basic Exercise Standards and Guidelines of the Aerobics and Fitness Association of America."

A. Definitions

1. Youth Fitness Programs

Youth fitness programs offer types of exercise which enhance the following components of fitness: flexibility, muscular strength and endurance, agility, balance, coordination, cardiovascular endurance and body composition. Movement patterns which help to develop motor skill and cognitive functions are also encouraged. Youth fitness does not necessarily imply that the activities are performed at a low intensity, as the intensity may vary according to age group and ability of each child. In addition, activity level depends on exercise selection, sequencing and movement patterns.

2. Growth

    Growth refers to changes in size, mea sured by weight and stature (height).

    a. Stages of postnatal growth:

        1) Infancy—the first year of life characterized by rapid growth of most bodily systems.

        2) Early childhood—1 to 5 years of age; a stage of rapid growth of trunk, lower extremities and large muscle groups.

        3) Middle childhood—6 to 10 years of age; a period of relatively steady progress in growth and maturation of all bodily functions.

        4) Prepubescent—children who have not developed secondary sex characteristics.

        5) Adolescence—8 to 19 years old in girls and 10 to 22 years old in boys; a period during which most bodily systems become mature in both structure and function. Structurally, adolescence begins with an acceleration in the rate of growth—commonly known as "growth spurt." Functionally, it is viewed as sexual maturation, beginning with an initial development of secondary sex characteristics and terminating with the attainment of mature reproductive function.

    b. Stature

        Stature, or height, is the most obvious difference between children and adults. Height is a consideration when: (1) expecting children to cover distance in a specified time (children take 2-3 times more steps to cover the same distance) and (2) changing levels, such as stepping up and down utilizing a bench or platform (platform height should be in proportion to child's leg length and physical ability).

3. Maturation

    Maturation refers to the process of growth and development which leads to achievement of adult characteristics. Maturation varies considerably among individuals and/or biological systems at any given age.

B. Importance of Physical Fitness and Movement

The promotion of physical activity in early and late childhood may be important in developing lifelong habits that may forestall future chronic illness, such as high blood pressure, elevated blood serum cholesterol, increased body fat, and heart disease. Early participation in physical activity has also demonstrated an increase in performance levels of fitness and motor skills. Numerous studies have supported the premise that important health and performance characteristics can be improved in children as a result of exercise.

The rationale for starting children on an exercise program at an early age includes, but is not limited to: (1) improved ability to meet the demands of daily physical activities; (2) improved results in physical performance tests; (3) improved motor skills; (4) reduced injuries; (5) fewer chronic health conditions and a lower risk for developing chronic health problems than sedentary children. In addition, physical activity has demonstrated development of: (1) self-esteem; (2) self-confidence; (3) responsibility; (4) social skills; (5) kinesthetic and spatial awareness; and (6) freedom of expression. Based on these important findings, children of all ages should be encouraged to be more physically active on a daily basis.

C. When Children Should Start Exercising

According to the American Academy of Pediatrics, "Guidelines for fitness and sports participation for preschool children younger than 6 years must be based on careful consideration of the physical fitness needs as well as the unique developmental requirements and limitations of this age group." Furthermore, it states, "There is no evidence that children's motor development can be accelerated or their subsequent sports performance influenced by physical training during the preschool years." Therefore, the following recommendations are suggested for **fitness programs for children younger than 6 years.**

1. All preschool children should participate in physical activity appropriate for their developmental level and physical health.

2. Goals for accelerating motor development to maximize later sports ability are inappropriate and futile.

3. Free play is preferable to structured exercise sessions in this age group.

4. Sports and fitness programs should be supervised by adults knowledgeable about the specific needs and limitations of preschool children.

5. Parents should serve as role models for children. Physical activities that parents can perform with young children should be encouraged.

D. Physical Ability vs. Chronological Age

1. First Skills Phase or Fundamental Movement Stage—2-5 years of age (preschool period): children begin to develop locomotion, stability and manipulation.

2. Basic Fitness Phase or Mature Stages of Fundamental Movement Phase—6-8 years of age

3. Early Team Phase—8-10 years of age: this is a transitional stage from fundamental movement to sports-related skills.

4. Sports Related Phase—10-14 years of age: children select specific sports or movement skills in which they wish to become proficient.

5. Specialized Movement Stage—14-17 years of age: a stage that represents the final choice of activities a child may tend to pursue in adulthood.

E. Instructor Qualifications

Instructors who are well-versed in child development and exercise and fitness concepts will have the leading edge when working with youth. They should maintain current instructor certification, CPR and advanced first aid. Certain states may require low-level FBI clearance and tuberculosis (TB) testing of instructors working with children, particularly for those working within the public school system. It is suggested that all fitness instructors inquire about such state regulations before beginning a youth program.

F. Role of Instructor

1. Instructors must be objective and flexible when teaching multiple age groups in order to offer effective and challenging programs.

2. Instructors must feel comfortable in their ability to work with children and be able to present fitness and play activities in a creative and innovative manner.

3. Instructors are often most successful when they: are able to think like a child; motivate and positively reinforce; serve as healthy and fit role models; set realistic goals; emphasize that all participants are winners; and provide a safe environment.

4. Instructors are encouraged to design a program that allows the children involved to participate in age-specific physical activity, encouraging personal best, in a structured, fun and non-competitive atmosphere.

G. Environmental Safety

To help ensure the safety of young fitness program participants, instructors are encouraged to follow the guidelines below.

1. Children should be supervised by you, the instructor, or another responsible adult at all times.

2. When working with very young children:

   a. Windows and storage cabinets should be locked when possible to prevent accidents.

   b. Electrical outlets should be covered.

3. Floors should be padded or, if not, use gym mats.

4. Lighting should be bright.

5. The exercise room should be free of sharp or obstructive objects.

6. All equipment, when not in use, should be properly stored.

H. Equipment

1. Equipment for children should be designed for the specific age group, according to size, material, weight, height and safety regulations.

2. Equipment for children should be: fun, safe, and quick and easy to store.

3. Young children love to use such props as: balls, balloons, hula hoops, feathers, hats, gloves and various costumes. Use your imagination. You might even ask the children what they enjoy playing with.

4. Creating homemade equipment, such as bean bags made from scraps of material or weights made from plastic bottles filled with water, can be a fun project for the children involved.

I. Music

1. Determine themes and use a variety of tunes.

2. Create an atmosphere through music selection.

3. Choose catchy melodies specific to certain age groups.

4. Utilize rhythms that are easy to move to.

5. Allow children to choose their favorite tunes.

II. Youth Fitness Endurance Training Principles and Guidelines (Age 6 through Adolescence)

Studies have demonstrated that children physiologically adapt to endurance training. Even though there is an abundance of literature citing the many benefits of aerobic exercise for children, the type, frequency, intensity and duration of exercise for optimal functional capacity and health have not been determined. Keep in mind youth fitness professionals may find it necessary to modify adult standards for establishing the intensity, duration and frequency of exercise for children ages 2-15. If you choose to use adult standards for principles of conditioning, these may be more appropriate for young people over the age of 15.

The following Guidelines are only recommendations, and should be modified according to the individual needs of the child.

A. Frequency

Youth fitness aerobic activities should be performed 2-3 times per week. As with all forms of cardiorespiratory conditioning, the response in children varies. Two to three days of endurance training should allow adequate time for participation in other activities, yet be sufficient enough to cause a training effect (ACSM, Rowland).

B. Duration

The attention span and physical capacity of children vary depending on their age and developmental stage. Therefore, it is important for the instructor to establish a specific amount of time appropriate for the chronological age and developmental level of his/her participants. For youth, duration of activity may be more beneficial than intensity due to the various developmental stages of maturation. A longer, less intense activity program may allow for a greater attention span with less physiological stress and provide positive health and social benefits.

For cardiorespiratory conditioning, when referring to adult norms, a class should include a minimum of 20 minutes and up to 45 minutes of aerobic activity within an individual's training heart rate range or rate of perceived exertion (RPE). An additional 3-10 minutes (3 minutes for preschool children and up to 10 minutes for adolescents) should be added for appropriate warm-up periods which include both rhythmic limbering movement and static stretching to facilitate range of motion development and injury prevention (see "Basic Exercise Standards and Guidelines," section V).

C. Intensity

As previously mentioned under duration, it is important for the instructor to establish an intensity level appropriate for the chronological age and developmental level of his/her participants.

To provide an aerobic training effect, an activity should provide sufficient overload to maintain a training heart rate. The aerobic portion should resemble a normal bell curve, as recommended for high-impact aerobics (see "Basic Exercise Standards and Guidelines," section VI.C). Intensity will vary depending on activity selected. Adult standards may be used to set and monitor the exercise intensity, but instructors should be aware of the limitations and controversies regarding their use (see section VI.A,1 of this chapter). It may be more appropriate to use 200 bpm minus age vs. 220 bpm minus age for estimated maximum heart rate (see section VI.A,1a of this chapter). Other ways to monitor exercise intensity may be used instead, such as the RPE scale. It is suggested that the RPE scale be modified for youth fitness programs so that it is easier to understand. For an aerobics class, exercise selection, elevated movement, movement patterns and sequencing, speed and lever length are important in regulating the exercise intensity.

Rate of Perceived Exertion Scale for Children		
Intensity	**Explanation**	**Visual example**
0-rest	How you feel when you are sitting and resting.	Child sitting in a chair or watching TV.
1-easy	How you feel when you are walking to school or doing chores around the house.	Child walking to school; no sweat.
2-pretty hard	How you feel when you are playing on the playground or running around.	Child playing and just starting to sweat.
3-harder	How you feel when you are playing on the playground or working hard.	Child playing sports and sweating.
4-hard	How you feel when you are running hard.	Child running hard and sweating profusely.
5-very hard, maximal	The hardest you have ever worked or exercised in your life.	Child running and ready to collapse at the finish line of a race.

(Reprinted with permission from Scott Roberts)

1. Activity Selection

   Children may achieve cardiorespiratory conditioning when participating in a variety of activities. See section III.B of this chapter.

2. Exercise Selection

   The variety of movements used and choice of exercise appropriate for the child's fitness level will be a determining factor in raising or lowering exercise intensity, as well as maintaining a consistent intensity level throughout the aerobic portion of the class. To determine the appropriate activities for a beginner, the instructor should design an activity questionnaire (see Appendix A of this chapter).

3. Speed of Movement

   See "Basic Exercise Standards and Guidelines," section I.F.

   The younger and less developed a child is, the slower his/her response time will be. Response time is divided into two components: (1) reaction time and (2) movement time. The instructor should be concerned with total response time in young children, making sure that demonstration of the desired movement pattern(s) is performed at a speed at which a young child can interpret and then perform.

Total response time will improve as one develops physically and chronologically up to the age of 20 years.

Length of arms and legs should also be considered when performing rhythmic limbering exercises. Children who have shorter limbs will move from side to center sooner than those with longer limbs. Therefore, variations in movement patterns and choreography should be applied according to the size of the participants and their physical abilities.

4. Muscle Strengthening

Muscular strengthening can be achieved in a youth fitness class without the use of added weight by the same methods utilized in traditional adult aerobic and body conditioning classes and with non-weighted floorwork (see "Basic Exercise Standards and Guidelines," sections V, VII and VIII). Factors to control include body position, muscle isolation, range of motion and repetitions.

5. Posture and Alignment

See "Basic Exercise Standards and Guidelines," section I.E, as well as alignment for specific body positions in sections V, VII, and VIII for muscle strengthening.

III. Class Format

Each program should be geared to a specific age group and defined by the cognitive, biomechanical and physiological capabilities of participants at each age level. Children between the ages of 2 and 5, and the ages of 6 and 8, respond more to programs emphasizing movement and play than specific fitness goals.

Individuals between age 9 and adulthood should participate in programs that emphasize the development of physical fitness components, such as: cardiovascular endurance, muscular strength and endurance, flexibility, balance, agility and coordination.

Design a program that will motivate children of all ages to develop positive, healthy, lifelong fitness habits.

A. Sequence

Class sequence for the older child (ages 16-18) who is participating in aerobic dance exercise will be the same as adult programming (see "Basic Exercise Standards and Guidelines," section II.A-C).

1. Pre-class Instruction

   a. Younger children have shorter attention spans than older children. Therefore, the time allotted for pre-class instruction should be adjusted according to the age and maturity level of the participants.

   b. From middle childhood to adolescence, teach how to take heart rate and the importance of monitoring heart rate during an exercise program.

c. Periodically reinforce proper breathing techniques and body alignment for all ages.

d. Include terminology and "real-life" examples that children are familiar with.

2. Warm-up

It is important to establish a habit of warming up the body prior to engaging in any strenuous activity. Therefore, children should be well-versed on the purpose of a warm-up. For the younger child whose attention span is short, a warm-up that is creative and fun is encouraged.

3. Aerobics Session

Youth fitness aerobics programming for cardiorespiratory conditioning may vary according to chronological age and maturity level of participants (see "Basic Exercise Standards and Guidelines," section VI.A-H). Keep in mind that modifications may need to be made in: the sequencing, speed and difficulty of movements, the height of steps or benches, and the type and size of playful props used with children.

4. Post-aerobic Cool-down

The purpose of the cool-down is to prevent blood from pooling in the lower extremities following aerobic exercise. Light activities during the cool-down may also help prevent muscle soreness.

5. Floorwork

Exercises from the following groups may be performed in order of preference: (a) legs, (b) buttocks, (c) hips, (d) abdominals and (e) lower back (see "Basic Exercise Standards and Guidelines," section II.A,4). The number of repetitions and intensity of movements should be reduced for youth fitness classes.

6. Cool-down Static Stretches

The purpose of the final cool-down static stretch is to increase the flexibility within the joints and return the body to a normal, relaxed state. See "Basic Exercise Standards and Guidelines," section XII.

B. **Types of Movement**

1. Ages 2-5

a. Focus on developing body awareness and responding to movement stimuli using music, sounds and equipment to help develop lateral movement skills, body control, balance, eye-hand coordination and body image.

b. To develop spatial awareness, visual perception and fundamental motor skills (gross motor and locomotive movements), utilize activities such as: climbing over, under, in and out, jumping, catching, falling, running, hopping, skipping, etc. Many of these activities may be incorporated into fun obstacle courses with colorful equipment and creative play set to music. Cognitive learning may be developed through the use of specific body parts, shapes, colors, etc.

c. Fantasy or make believe movement adventures encourage children to explore a wide range of movement patterns in a continuous, creative and fun manner.

d. Children move with intermittent bursts of energy. Therefore, classes should be well supervised, yet loosely structured and designed to follow children's natural movement patterns.

e. Sample class format

Class Length:	20-40	minutes
Pre-class Instruction: (including health/fitness tips)	3-5	minutes
Warm-up:	3-5	minutes
Activity Session:	15-20	minutes
Cool-down:	3-5	minutes
Closure (award system):	3-5	minutes

(See section X.B of this chapter.)

2. Ages 6-8

a. Focus on increased body awareness, rhythm and coordination, music memory, further development of motor skills, and eye-hand coordination. A circuit format is ideal for this age group since attention span is short. The circuit should include a variety of different exercise stations to challenge the individual, help increase awareness and isolate different body parts.

b. Group activities which include multi-impact movement combinations to help develop rhythm and muscle memory as well as group cooperative games are encouraged. This age group can also benefit from more complex obstacle courses which incorporate the use of large muscles, locomotive skills, visual perception, spatial awareness, and cognitive and motor functions.

c. Introduce participants to basic sports skills.

d. Introduce kids' step and slide programs.

e. Sample class format

Class Length:	45-60	minutes
Pre-class Instruction: (including health/fitness tips)	5	minutes
Warm-up:	5-10	minutes
Activity Session:	25-30	minutes
Cool-down:	5-10	minutes
Closure (award system):	5	minutes

3. Ages 9-11

a. Design a program that will increase physical skills. For example: a circuit which combines movement sequences, cardiovascular conditioning, muscle strength and endurance, flexibility, agility and balance.

b. Cooperative games may be incorporated to enhance social skills and group play (sportsmanship).

c. Continue instruction for basic sports skills.

d. Introduce fun, creative, low-impact aerobic dance exercise. Instructor may also choose to introduce children to kids' step and slide programs.

e. Introduce strength training. Teach proper technique and form using natural resistance and light weights (1/2-1 pound).

f. Sample class format

Class Length:	45-60 minutes
Pre-class Instruction: (including health/fitness tips)	5 minutes
Warm-up:	5-10 minutes
Aerobic Conditioning:	20 minutes
Post-aerobic Cool-down:	5 minutes
Strengthening:	10-15 minutes
Final Cool-down:	3-5 minutes

4. Ages 12-15

a. Focus on exercises that stress the components of physical fitness: cardiovascular endurance, muscular strength and endurance, flexibility, agility and balance.

b. The use of circuits and advanced obstacle courses is appropriate.

c. All related sports, both individual and team, are of particular interest to this age group. Instructors may focus on developing sports skills.

d. Introduce more challenging movement patterns for low-impact aerobic dance.

e. Continue instruction in strength training (see section VIII of this chapter).

f. Gradually increase intensity and duration of aerobic portion of class until minimum adult standards are met (see "Basic Exercise Standards and Guidelines," section VI).

g. Keep students moving to burn calories.

h. See section III.B,3e of this chapter for sample class format.

5. Ages 16-18

a. See section III.B,4a-g of this chapter.

b. Instructors may choose to focus on advanced skills and play strategies for individual and team athletic sports.

c. Instruction in aerobic dance exercise, funk, step and slide (if equipment is available) may be incorporated in a program designed for this age group.

d. For class format, see section III.B,3e of this chapter and "Basic Exercise Standards and Guidelines," section II.

IV. Pre-Class Procedure

A. Instructor Checklist

Review points to cover in "Basic Exercise Standards and Guidelines," sections III-IV. Because children are not able to give legal consent, parents must sign a permission or consent form before children should be allowed to participate in youth fitness classes. Instructors should take the following steps before children are allowed to exercise.

1. Verify that medical clearance has been obtained.
2. Determine the appropriate level of participation.
3. Ensure appropriate shoes are being worn.
4. Instruct the child how to breathe properly during exercise.
5. Give an aerobic class orientation. An instructor may wish to include a description of and directions for the day's activities, a special healthy thought in regard to aerobic fitness, the reward for the day if one is being given, etc.
6. Determine and explain the training heart rate and perceived exertion levels.
7. Review safety procedures.

B. Youth Fitness Orientation

Familiarize youth participants with important body alignment cues for maintaining proper positioning and receiving optimal fitness benefits from their workout. You may choose to repeat these cues often throughout the program. Review the following important points, using demonstration if necessary.

1. Complete all movements through the full range of motion.
2. Control the speed of movements.
3. Use arms, legs and feet during combinations and movement patterns to maintain workout intensity.

V. Warm-Up (Middle Childhood through Adolescence)

A. Purpose

To prepare the body for vigorous exercise and reduce the risk of injury (see "Basic Exercise Standards and Guidelines," section V.A).

B. Time

Class should always begin with a 5-10 minute warm-up, including exercises specific to muscles that will be utilized during the workout. Some studies have shown that children do not need as lengthy a warm-up as adults.

C. Specific Warm-up Guidelines

The guidelines for static stretching, warm-up sequence, muscle groups, rhythmic limbering exercises and special do's and don'ts, as described in the "Basic Exercise Standards and Guidelines," section V, should be followed for a youth fitness class.

VI. Cardiorespiratory Conditioning without Weights (Middle Childhood through Adolescence)

A. Purpose

To train the cardiovascular and respiratory systems to exchange and deliver oxygen quickly and efficiently to each part of the body being exercised.

1. Special Concerns

   a. Aerobic capacity-a prepubescent child's maximum capacity for oxygen utilization (VO_2 max) averages 1 liter per minute compared to 3 liters per minute for a 21-year-old. A 7-year-old boy has approximately 1/4 the muscle mass of an adult male. This difference in size is the primary reason for the variance in aerobic capacity between adults and children. Due to this reduced work capacity in children, adult norms should be adjusted accordingly for aerobic activities when programming youth fitness.

   b. Children's capacity for anaerobic exercise is also dramatically reduced due to size, growth and development. Therefore, fatigue may occur sooner than expected during high-intensity activities. Intersperse anaerobic activities with breaks to enable the children to rest and hydrate.

   c. Children have increased ventilatory rates due to smaller lungs.

B. Time

20-45 minutes, not including warm-up or post-aerobic cool-down.

C. Sequence

Start slowly, gradually increasing the intensity and range of motion of your movements. All considerations discussed in the "Basic Exercise Standards and Guidelines," section VI.A-J, should be adhered to until such a time when a steady state has been achieved, approximately 3-5 minutes after the aerobic portion has begun. Heart rate in youth fitness programs should be maintained in the 55-80% range of estimated maximum heart rate.

See "Basic Exercise Standards and Guidelines," section VI.I for calculation and monitoring methods. For early to middle childhood, monitoring exercise through perceived exertion may be more appropriate. For the adolescent, a combination of perceived exertion and pulse taking is recommended. Heart rate calculations may be more effective when using a maximum heart rate of 200 versus 220 (Rowland, 1990). Heart rate may be elevated or decreased by regulating the intensity of the exercises. Factors affecting intensity can be found in section II.C of this chapter.

VII. Post-Aerobic Cool-Down (Middle Childhood through Adolescence)

A. Purpose

To provide a transition period between vigorous aerobic work and less taxing exercise, thus allowing working heart rate to safely return to pre-exercise rate without overstressing cardiorespiratory function. Children seem to recover from exercise faster than adults.

B. Time

2-5 minutes.

C. Type of Movement

Rhythmic movement that gradually decreases in speed and range of motion.

D. Method

Proceed with 2-5 minutes of rhythmic movement, followed by static stretching for the back, shoulders and arms, as well as calves, quadriceps, hamstrings and front of shins. Check heart rate either by perceived exertion or pulse. Heart rate should be 60% or less of estimated maximum heart rate before beginning the floorwork. If specific arm work has not been accomplished either during or prior to the aerobic section, proceed with post-aerobic cool-down described above, followed by specific arm work, according to "Basic Exercise Standards and Guidelines," section V.A-F. Conclude with static stretching and heart rate check as described below.

VIII. Major Muscle Conditioning

See "Basic Exercise Standards and Guidelines," sections VIII-XI. The number of repetitions may need to be appropriately adjusted for different age groups and various fitness levels. Begin muscle strengthening programs with slow, progressive stages, starting with 5-8 repetitions and gradually increasing the repetitions as children become more proficient and ready for a challenge. The instructor's role is to try to avoid risk of injury to his/her young, developing participants.

IX. Resistance Training Guidelines and Recommendations

A. Introduction and Recommendations

The issue of children lifting weights was not widely accepted until recently. Early investigators led many to believe that strength gains were not even possible in prepubescent children, and strength training could cause irreversible injury to the developing growth plates in bones. However, despite the fact that there are fewer resistance training studies involving children than adults, there is now substantial evidence demonstrating voluntary increases in strength following structured resistance training in children. These increases are similar to those observed in older age groups. Furthermore, the safety and efficacy of resistance training programs for prepubescent children have been well documented.

In addition to improvements in muscular strength, other fitness and performance related effects of resistance training include: (1) increased flexibility, (2) improved physical performance, (3) improved body composition, (4) improved cardiorespiratory fitness, (5) reduced serum lipids and (6) reduced blood pressure. With further research, additional benefits may be realized.

For further information, see "Basic Exercise Standards and Guidelines for Weighted Workouts."

1. Resistance Training

   Children should be encouraged to participate in a variety of activities that involve repetitive movements against an opposing force.

2. Free Weight Training

   Proper lifting techniques and safety are the two most important factors to consider. Start with small 1/2- to 1-pound dumbbells. Perform a variety of upper and lower body exercises.

3. Weight Training Machines

   With the exception of several companies which manufacture weight training equipment specifically for children, most exercise equipment is designed for adults. If children cannot be properly fitted for the machines, do not use them.

4. Manual Resistance Training

   With manual resistance training, resistance is provided by a partner. Children take turns applying resistance during different movements. For example, to perform hip abduction one child lies on the ground while the other child applies resistance to the leg being raised (abducted). Caution should be taken while performing partner resistant or stretching exercises. Make sure the children are at a psychological maturity level to understand the importance of performing correct technique and potential risk for injury (age 10 and up).

5. Isometric Training

   Isometric training occurs when muscles are contracted but do not change in length. For example, to perform standing upright lateral raises one child tries to raise his/her arms up and out to the sides while the other child applies the resistant force at the upper arms (partner work). Isometric exercises can also be done individually.

6. Tubing Exercises

   Exercise tubing can be purchased or made from scratch in different levels of resistance. All resistance exercises should be performed in a slow, steady, sustained manner. Use a specific count during the initial movement, the hold phase and then return to the resting phase.

7. Additional Programs

To perform pulling activities, tie a rope to a wall and have the children pull themselves toward the wall while sitting on a piece of carpet; or they may pull weighted sandbags toward themselves. Pushing activities include push-ups and throwing a medicine ball.

For hanging activities, the child may hang from a bar, swing, or slowly release from an assisted pull-up (eccentric work).

8. Strengthening Without the Use of Weights

If strengthening exercises without weights are to be included for the upper and lower body (arms, chest, shoulders, back and/or legs, buttocks and abdominals), see "Basic Exercise Standards and Guidelines," sections VIII-XII.

B. Specific Guidelines

Studies have shown that individuals between the ages of 10 and 19 are particularly prone to injury during strength training. This may be due to the fact that bones are still developing (see section X.A,1-2 of this chapter). It also may be associated with children lifting maximal weights and performing improper lifting techniques (Kraemer & Fleck, 1993). However, most of these injuries occur at home or during non-supervised activity. Generally, strength training machines and isokinetic devices are considered safer than free weights for young people over the age of 14. Most children (ages 6-8) and adolescents can develop adequate strength and endurance with calisthenic exercises (see "Basic Exercise Standards and Guidelines," sections VIII-XII), gymnastics, and activities such as swimming and wrestling.

1. The following precautions should be taken with children when they participate in a strength training program.

   a. Children should be at such a level of emotional and physical maturity that they can understand and follow specific rules and instructional procedures.

   b. Exercises should be fun and non-competitive in a group situation. Competition *is* acceptable on an individual level when a child is seeking self-improvement and can be rewarded by his/her own personal drive, self-esteem and goal setting.

   c. Emphasize higher repetitions and sets (12-16 reps, 2-4 sets) and less weight. Lifting heavier weights depends on the child's individual maturation level and training experience.

   d. Lifting maximal, or near-maximal, resistance (less than 6 reps) is not recommended during a child's developmental years. Injuries may occur related to the long bones and the back.

   e. Supervision by competent instructors is very important.

   f. The instructor should teach proper warm-up and stretching techniques prior to lifting weights.

   g. Children and adolescents should learn to perform a variety of calisthenic and strength training exercises.

h. Children should learn the purpose of performing each exercise and how to combine them into a logical sequence or progression.

i. Strength training should be part of a complete fitness program which includes cardiovascular fitness, flexibility and a well-balanced diet.

j. Encourage children to keep track of their progress through the use of logs, charts, creative maps, etc.

2. The following "Basic Guidelines for Resistance Exercise Progression in Children" was written by William J. Kraemer, Ph.D. and Steven J. Fleck, Ph.D., authors of *Strength Training for Young Athletes.*

a. Age 7 or younger—Introduce child to basic exercises with little or no weight (see "Basic Exercise Standards and Guidelines," section VIII-XI). Develop the concept of a training session. Teach exercise techniques, progressing from body weight calisthenics to partner exercises and lightly resisted exercises. Keep volume (a measure of the total work-sets x repetitions x resistance for a given exercise, training session or training period) low.

b. Ages 8-10—Gradually increase the number of exercises. Practice technique in all lifts. Start gradual progressive loading of exercises (see "Basic Exercise Standards and Guidelines for Weighted Workouts"). Keep exercises simple. Gradually increase volume. Carefully monitor toleration to the exercise stress.

c. Ages 11-13—Teach all basic exercise techniques. Continue progressive loading of each exercise, emphasizing techniques. Introduce more advanced exercises with little or no resistance.

d. Ages 14-15—Progress to more advanced youth programs in resistance exercise. Add sport-specific components, emphasizing exercise techniques and increasing volume.

e. Age 16 and older—Move child to entry-level adult programs after all background knowledge has been mastered and a basic level of training experience has been gained.

Note: Gradually introduce a child to a resistance training program by slowly progressing to more advanced levels as exercise toleration, skill, amount of training time and understanding permit.

X. Special Considerations Related to Youth Fitness

A. Growth and Development Issues

1. Activity increases skeletal growth. For example, vigorous activity may affect the bone structure and strength, thus creating more resistance to injury.

2. The growth plates do not fuse until maturity when hardening of the bones occurs (which may not be until ages 18-20 years). Maturation of the skeletal system occurs at different rates in different individuals. There may be a 5- to 6-year difference between chronological age and skeletal maturity.

3. In children, muscular strength develops concurrent with chronological development.

4. Lean body weight is the most important factor in the development of strength and power in children.

5. Many experts profess that physical activity begun and consistently performed in childhood has an impact on the child's body and activity level throughout life.

6. As children mature, their responses to training improve. Both strength and maximal oxygen uptake are strongly related to the proportion of lean body mass in developing children.

7. The degree to which children can improve physiological measures depends on growth and maturation rates and the exercise stimulus during exercise training.

B. Psychological Issues

Unlike adults, young children will not exercise when fatigued for the sake of health, beauty or fitness. Motivation levels differ between adults, teens and children. Though extrinsic motivators should not be relied upon too heavily, it may be necessary to provide tangible reinforcers, such as stars, stickers, certificates, etc., to help motivate the younger child. These reinforcers should be linked with praise. With age, tangible reinforcers may be diminished as children become more intrinsically motivated. Keep in mind that people of all ages need praise, recognition and positive motivational tips from fitness professionals.

C. Medical Issues

1. Asthma

   Approximately 4 million children are affected by asthma in the United States. The National Heart, Lung and Blood Institute recommends that children with asthma exercise when they are feeling well. Start slowly and gradually build into an exercise program. Consult with parents and physician prior to starting a child on any exercise program.

2. Diabetes

   It is recommended to encourage children with controlled diabetes to exercise. Participation in regular exercise helps to expend energy, reduce body fat and improve diabetic control. Instructors should be well versed on diabetes, its symptoms, treatment and emergency protocol. A signed release from the child's physician and parents should be obtained before starting an exercise program.

3. Obesity

   The benefits of regular exercise participation for the obese child are not limited to weight loss. Other benefits of exercise for these children include reduction in blood serum cholesterol and blood pressure and an increase in positive self-image. Lead the obese child through a slow, progressive exercise program to ensure continual participation. Refer to "Exercise Standards and Guidelines for the Overweight Participant."

XI. Injury Prevention

A. Research indicates children tolerate increases in workloads equal to adults, but modified for height and size.

B. Physiological factors influence children exercising during hot weather. Children have:

1. Higher surface area/mass ratios.

2. Greater amount of heat transfer between the body and environment.

3. Greater metabolic heat production than adults performing the same activity.

4. Less sweating capacity than adults.

5. Decreased ability to get rid of heat, due to lowered cardiac output and size.

C. **Hot Weather Precautions**

1. Monitor temperature and humidity and adjust activities accordingly.

2. Until adaptation occurs, children acclimating to hot temperatures should use a gradual approach to strenuous fitness programs. Instructors should be aware that children tend to have a 20-30% greater energy expenditure than adults during aerobic activities. This coupled with lower sweat rates, lower cardiac output and greater surface area to mass ratio can impair temperature regulation. Children should drink water frequently and exercise for less than 30 minutes in temperatures over 85° Fahrenheit.

3. Children should be encouraged to drink cool fluids prior to, during and after activity. Cool water is recommended over other fluids, such as juice, soda, Gatorade, etc. Avoid fluids with caffeine as these can promote dehydration.

4. Children should wear a lightweight, single layer of absorbent material so sweat evaporation is facilitated.

5. The American Academy of Pediatrics Committee on Sports Medicine has identified children with the following conditions to be at high risk for heat stress problems.

   - Obesity

   - Fevers of sweating syndrome

   - Cystic fibrosis, gastrointestinal infections, diabetes insipidus, diabetes mellitus, chronic heart failure, malnutrition, anorexia nervosa and mental deficiency.

D. **Distance Running and Children**

The International Athletics Association Federation Medical Committee states the following about distance running and children. "The danger certainly exists that with over-intensive training, separation of the growth plates may occur in the pelvic region, the knee or the ankle." In fact, the Committee recommends that children under 12 years of age run no more than a 1/2 mile in competition.

E. Most Common Childhood Injuries

1. Cuts, bruises and scrapes
2. Joint sprains
3. Muscular strains
4. Fractures

F. To help ensure against injury during exercise, it is suggested that children:

1. Have thorough physical exams before pursuing an exercise program.
2. Be cautioned about abruptly increasing the intensity, duration or frequency of exercise.
3. Participate in a warm-up and cool-down.
4. Perform flexibility exercises following a brief cardiovascular warm-up.
5. Wear proper clothing and footwear.
6. Exercise in a safe environment. Be aware of spacing, floor surfaces, lighting, ventilation, foreign objects, etc. Program should be well supervised, with children aware of specific rules and regulations.
7. Stop exercising if they feel dizzy, lightheaded, nauseous, pain, etc. (see "Basic Exercise Standards and Guidelines," III.A.2.b.)

G. Emergency Protocol

1. First-aid Technique
   a. Instructors are encouraged to remain current on immediate first-aid procedures so they are able to deal effectively with emergencies.
   b. Have an emergency game plan so you know who to call, how to call and what to do in case of serious injury.
   c. Know and practice CPR.
   d. Practice RICE—Rest, Ice, Compression and Elevation
   e. Know the essentials of wound care (see appendix A of *Fitness: Theory and Practice*, AFAA, 1995):
      1) Stop the bleeding.
      2) Cleanse the wound.
      3) Protect the wound.
      4) Treat for shock.

2. First-aid Materials

   A comprehensive first-aid kit for the treatment of injuries should be easily accessible to instructors. Check to make sure your kit and facility have the following materials.

   a. Ice, ice chest and plastic bags

b. Elastic bandages of varying widths

c. Soap or antiseptic

d. Bandages and gauze

e. Band-Aids

f. Splinting material

g. Sling

h. Clean water

i. Athletic tape

j. Scissors

k. Syrup of Ipecac

l. Smelling salts

m. Rubber gloves

n. Mask for CPR

H. Miscellaneous

1. Discipline/Control

    Be consistent in managing discipline and enforcing rules. Younger children who are acting out of control may be asked to:

    a. Take a "time-out" (designate a safe and supervised space in the exercise room for "time-outs").

    b. Receive pre-established consequences after initial warnings.

2. Encourage parents to participate in their child's fitness program when appropriate. This can reinforce (a) family togetherness, (b) parent as active role model and (c) a further involvement in family activities.

3. Competition vs. Cooperation

    a. Cooperative sports and activities help to develop social skills both physically and emotionally (e.g., respect for others, sportsmanship, communication and team-play).

    b. Competitive sports and activities can promote positive self-esteem and an inner drive to reach one's potential. However, competitive sports and competition in general may not be for everyone and could actually have a negative effect on children who are unprepared physically and/or emotionally for this type of environment.

References

American Academy of Pediatrics (1983). Weight training and weightlifiting: Information for the pediatrician. *The Physician and Sports Medicine*, 11: 157-161.

American Fitness Magazine (July/August, 1991). Special youth fitness section. *American Fitness*, 23-30.

Antonacci, R.J., & Barr, J. (1975). *Physical fitness for young champions* (2nd ed.). San Francisco: McGraw Hill Co.

Bar-Or, O. (1984). Trainability of the prepubescent child. *The Physician and Sports Medicine*, 5: 64-82.

Holland, M. (March 24-28, 1993). Fitness and play for kids: Designing programs for all ages. (Lecture). IRSA convention, San Diego, Ca.

Journal of Physical Education, Recreation and Dance (JOPHERD) (May/June, 1993). Dance dynamics: Dance education K-12-theory into practice, part III. *JOPHERD*, 41-59.

Journal Physical Education, Recreation and Dance (JOPHERD) (October, 1993). Leisure today: Leisure programming: The state of the art. *JOPHERD*, 25-51.

Kraemer, W.J., & Fleck, S.J. (1993). *Strength training for young athletes*. Champaign, Ill.: Human Kinetics Publishers, Inc.

Nichols, M. (1993). California School of Fitness, San Diego, Ca.

Pangrazi, R.P., & Corbin, C.B. (September, 1993). Physical fitness: Questions teachers ask. *Journal of Physical Education, Recreation and Dance*, 14-19.

Pemberton, C.L., & McSwegin, P.J. (May/June, 1993). Sedentary living: A health hazard. *Journal of Physical Education, Recreation and Dance*, 72-75.

Pica, R. (May/June, 1993). Responsibility and young children: What does physical education have to do with it? *Journal of Physical Education, Recreation and Dance*, 72-75.

Reebok, Instructor News (1992). Family fitness. Dallas: The Cooper Institute for Aerobics Research, 5: 4.

Roberts, S.O. (1993). Exercise quidelines for children. In *Fitness: Theory & Practice*. Sherman Oaks, Ca.: Aerobics and Fitness Association of America, 379-382.

Roberts, S.O., & Weider, B. (in press). The strength and weight training guide for young athletes. Chicago, Ill.: Contemporary Books.

Rowland, T.W. (1990). *Exercise and children's health*. Champaign, Ill.: Human Kinetics Publishers, Inc.

Sallis, J.F., et al. (1992). Determination of physical activity and interventions in youth. *Medicine and Science in Sports and Exercise*, 24:6: S248-S257.

Saris, W.H.M. (1985). The assessment and evaluation of daily physical activity in children. A review. *Acta Pediatric Scandinavia*, 318: 37-48.

Seefeldt, V. (November/December, 1984). Physical fitness in preschool and elementary school-aged children. *Journal of Health, Physical Education, Recreation and Dance*, 33-40.

Seefeldt, V. (1993). Personal interview. Youth Sports Institute, Lansing, Mi.

Wood, A. (1986). Aerobic dance for children: Resources and recommendations. *Physician and Sportsmedicine*, 14: 3.

Appendix A

NAME_____

Physical Activity Questionnaire

Parents: please complete the following questionnaire concerning your child.

1. During the past few months, what would best describe your child's usual level of physical acitvity? (circle one)
   a. Inactive-watches TV, reads or does homework after school; takes bus or gets ride to school; does not participate in any extracurricular sports.
   b. Occasionally Active-prefers sedentary activities, but sometimes plays outside.
   c. Moderately Active-takes opportunities to become involved in physical activity when available and enjoys it.
   d. Active-takes initiative to participate in physical exercise and prefers this to sedentary activities. Gets involved in vigorous exercise at least three times per week.
   e. Very Active-regularly participates in extracurricular sports. Has a great deal of energy. Dislikes sedentary activities.

2. How would you compare the physical activity of your child with that of his/her friends? (check one)
   ❑ Equally active   ❑ More active   ❑ Less active

3. During the past six months was your child involved in an organized sport or exercise program (such as YMCA, basketball league, gymnastics, dancing lessons) outside of regular school physical education?
   ❑ Yes, describe:_____
   ❑ No

4. During the last six months was your child regularly involved in athletic training (running, bicycling, swiming, etc.)?
   ❑ Yes   ❑ No

5. In your opinion, is your child as physically active as she/he should be? (check one)
   ❑ Yes   ❑ Too active   ❑ Not active enough

6. If you feel your child is not sufficiently active, what do you feel is the reason? (check all that apply)
   ❑ Not interested   ❑ Doesn't feel talented in sports   ❑ Too busy
   ❑ Illness   ❑ Exercise in uncomfortable   ❑ Friends aren't interested
   Other reason(s):_____

7. How much time per day would you estimate your child spends being physically active (running, playing outside, sports, etc.)? ____hours. And how many hours does he/she spend being sedentary (watching Tv, reading, etc.)? ____hours.

8. Do you feel your child's school provides adequate instruction in physical education and health education?
   ❑ Yes   ❑ No

9. How many hours per week do you (parent) participate in regular physical fitness activities? ____hours.

10. List the different kinds of physical activities your family does together (walking, hiking, playing, etc.).

    _____

    _____

Reprinted with permission from Scott Roberts.

Part III

Exercise Modality

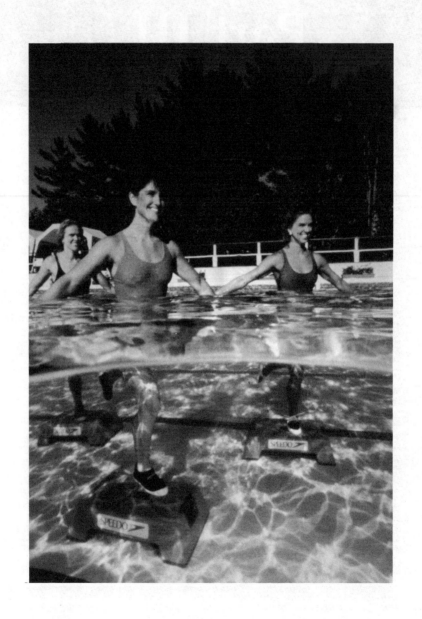

STANDARDS AND GUIDELINES

of the

Aerobics and Fitness Association of America

for

Basic Water Exercise/Aqua Fitness

Since land and water exercises are different, these guidelines are written to target the unique water environment and how it affects standard exercise science principles. These guidelines do not serve as a training, but provide research-based information to apply to water exercise programs for optimal training. To understand how water affects the body during exercise, it is essential for the instructor to evaluate movements in the water. These guidelines should be applied to practical water-application exercises to evaluate their safety and water-specific function.

These guidelines are written to accompany AFAA's Basic Exercise Standards and Guidelines written for land exercise with consideration of the water environment. This information references the land exercise principles and simply addresses the application of land exercise principles to the unique environment of water.

These guidelines are written for the "healthy," average, asymptomatic population, who is seeking improvements in cardiovascular endurance, muscular strength/endurance, flexibility and body composition for general health and are intended to be used in conjunction with AFAA's "Basic Exercise Standards and Guidelines."

Introduction

Water exercise is becoming more popular as a fitness choice. In order to optimize training, every movement must be designed according to the water's effect against the body. The two primary effects are resistance and buoyancy. As Carol Kennedy, M.S., exercise physiologist at Indiana University says, "the exercises should be purposeful and your students should understand why they are performing them."

The environment of water is different than land. If your task were to design an exercise program for outer space, you would need to examine the effect of anti-gravity environment on the body and determine what movements create training. The same is true for water. Gravity still affects the body, however, the degree varies with a number of conditions. Since the viscosity of water is greater than air, resistance to movement is greater in water creating the opportunity to make an easy movement more difficult. Keep in mind, however, the effects of buoyancy on the body provide the opportunity to make movements easier.

In order to design functional training movements, consideration must be given to the following:

A. Water's properties acting on the body.

B. Application of standardized guidelines for land exercise supported by current research and accepted industry methods.

C. Exercise designs that combine the properties of water, land exercise science and current scientific water research to create functional "water-specific" movements that improve health and fitness levels.

Poorly designed water exercises may not create an appropriate intensity to fall within the recommended guidelines for training and fitness results may not be optimized. To become a good technician and exercise designer, the water environment must be examined to understand the difference of its effect, both when a body is submerged and when a body is moving through it. Land-based exercise science principles learned from years of research can be applied to the water environment to create a new type of training. These new methods require basic skills which must be learned for successful training results to occur. For a person to be able to swim for fitness, they must first learn how to swim! Water fitness skills are not as complicated as swimming. However, without some basic skills, it's difficult to achieve a training intensity. Basic fundamental skills, when mastered, can provide the opportunity for people to take responsibility for regulating their own work intensity. This establishes the foundation for a variety of unique water movements or programs that can be included in a lifestyle fitness program.

Key terms

ACSM—the American College of Sports Medicine.

Calisthenics—stationary exercises such as standing leg lifts and push-ups that are designed to build flexibility, muscular strength and endurance and condition specific muscle groups.

Cardiovascular endurance—includes conditioning of the heart and lungs for an aerobic, cardiovascular training effect. This type of exercise improves the efficacy of the heart and lungs, and the ability of the body to meet the skeletal demands for oxygen. Oxygen consumption or VO_2 max measure the ability of the body to maximize oxygen uptake and describe the arterial venous difference which is an indicator of cardiovascular endurance capacity.

Deep water—water depth measured on an individual "standing" in a vertical position when the lungs are submerged-usually about armpit depth and deeper. At this depth, the feet may be touching the bottom lightly or not at all.

Flexibility—refers to the range of motion in a joint or groups of joints.

Intensity progression—a method of increasing or decreasing workload by varying a component of a move to gradually change the degree or level of physical difficulty.

Muscular condition—the combination of muscular strength and endurance.

Muscular strength—the ability of muscle to exert force, usually measured as the maximum load that can be lifted once. Training for this component includes high loads and low repetitions.

Muscular endurance—the ability to contract repeatedly with the same force over an extended period of time, usually measured by the number of repetitions performed at a low load until muscles fatigue. Although weak muscles may not be able to sustain activities for a long period of time, greater muscular strength can support muscular endurance by helping to resist fatigue.

Properties of water—the unique characteristics of water that affect the body during exercise in water including inertia, buoyancy, resistance and action/reaction.

    a.   Inertia—force must be applied to move a body from rest, stop a moving body or change the direction of a moving body. Inertia is the resistance to change.

    b.   Buoyancy—Archimedes' Principle of buoyancy states that when a body is partially or wholly immersed in any fluid, it experiences an upward thrust equal to the weight of fluid displaced.

    c.   Resistance—resistance varies with a number of conditions. Drag resistance or form drag relates to the surface area (shape and lever length) and smoothness of the object moving through the water. Drag force acts to oppose motion and will increase as the size of surface area and speed of the surface increases. Surface area and speed must be considered when evaluating their effect on resistance against the body during exercise.

    d.   Action/Reaction—Newton's law states for every action there is an equal and opposite reaction.

Shallow water—navel to nipple depth measured with the individual standing on the bottom of the pool.

Shallow water calisthenics—stationary movements performed in shallow water involving variations in lever (arm and leg) actions which focus on training individual muscle groups. Movements are performed primarily "on the beat" for a specific number of repetitions.

Shallow water rhythmic exercises—movements performed in shallow water in either a stationary or traveling mode. Utilizing a variety of muscle groups and cadences, they involve a number of movement sizes (large and small). Movements are paced by intensity progressions during a training time period without regard to the number of repetitions performed at a specific beat.

Thermal regulation—maintenance of core body temperature by establishing a balance between metabolic heat production and heat loss.

Water comfort—the ability to relax and move freely through water in a vertical position without fear or panic.

Water fitness or water exercise—exercises performed primarily in a vertical orientation in shallow or deep water. This type of exercise program usually does not include swimming skills, which are based on efficient propulsion horizontally through the water. Water exercise instead uses movements that amplify drag by unstreamlining the body to create resistance. The goal of this water-based program is to create sufficient intensity to provide fitness training adaptations in oxygen consumption (V0$_2$ max), muscular strength, endurance, flexibility and body composition.

Water-specific—movements, exercises or equipment designed to amplify the properties of water by manipulating the water's effect on the body.

I. Basic Principles, Definitions and Recommendations

A. Components of Physical Fitness

The four health-related components of physical fitness are addressed in water exercise programs. Targeting the training zone with specific water exercise design is different. However, the goals for health are the same.

1. Cardiovascular efficiency and endurance: Research shows single bouts of water exercise can improve cardiovascular endurance with average VO_2 falling within the range recommended by the American College of Sports Medicine (ACSM) (Cassady, 1992; Johnson, 1977; Heberlein et al., 1992). This predicted response is supported with a number of long-term, training adaptation studies which report significant improvements in cardiovascular fitness during programs in shallow and deep water (Barretta, 1993; Hoeger et al., 1993; Michaud, et al, 1992; Ruoti, 1994; Sanders, 1993; Stevenson, 1988). Some programs fail to report significant improvements and will be examined under "Specificity of Training" to determine why.

2. Muscular Strength and Endurance: The ACSM recommends at least 2 sessions of resistance training per week. The water's viscosity provides resistance with every movement, making it a resistive environment. Improvements in this area can only be measured by research studies which focus on resistance training using water as the resistance. Several studies found significant improvements in muscular strength/endurance for the upper and lower body as well as the trunk (Barretta, 1993; Hoeger, 1993; Sanders, 1993; Ruoti, 1994). In Hoeger's (1993) study, shallow water rhythmic exercise produced greater muscular strength improvements than a low-impact aerobics class. Sanders (1993) found significant gains in abdominal endurance without using a typical "crunch" type exercise during the program. The gains are thought to be a result of dynamic postural alignment while traveling through the water.

3. Flexibility: Flexibility gains for the lower back and hamstrings are supported by research studies (Hoeger, 1993; Miss, 1988; Barretta, 1993). However, other studies contradict these results. Further investigation of the methods used to achieve these gains needs to be conducted.

4. Optimal Body Composition: Unfortunately, much of the widely publicized research in water was conducted on swimmers and reported either no fat loss or an increase in body fat (Gwinup, 1987; Stavish, 1987). The results of rhythmic water exercise studies indicate significant improvements in body composition which are similar to land exercise training programs (Abraham, 1994; Barretta, 1993; Hoeger, 1993; Knecht, 1989; Sanders, 1993).

B. Principles of Training

1. Training Effect

   The training effect in water is the same with consideration given to appropriate frequency, intensity and duration, and training should be (1) consistent, (2) progressive and (3) specific. A training effect will occur if the exercise is sufficient in all of the following areas:

a. frequency: number of exercise days per week

b. intensity: degree of physical stress

c. duration: length of time.

Due to buoyancy, impact in water is decreased. Participants can regulate their intensity by simply slowing down while continuing the work. This creates active rest phases as needed "on demand." This instant regulation of intensity may allow a student to extend the period of time spent exercising in water when compared to a program performed on land using constant forces of gravity. Less impact may also make it possible to exercise more frequently without increasing the risk for overuse injury. By developing rest/work skills, some people may increase their total exercise time thereby contributing to a higher level of activity and greater calorie expenditure during the week, month and year.

2. Overload Principle

In water, the exercise principle of "overload" applies the same as on land. How this principle is applied will be addressed later (see "Basic Exercise Standards and Guidelines," II.B.2.).

3. Specificity of Training

Targeting training for each of the components of fitness is the same in water as on land. How we target training in water is different and is covered under applications (see "Basic Exercise Standards and Guidelines," I.B.3.).

4. Mode of exercise in this article refers only to water-based programs. These programs may be formatted in a number of ways to target types of training, such as cardiovascular endurance or muscular strength/endurance. Various types of exercise workouts may include intervals, continuous, muscular endurance work using high number of repetitions or flexibility work that targets stretching.

C. **Frequency of aerobic training** (Refer to I.C., Frequency of Aerobic Training, "Basic Exercise Standards and Guidelines").

1. Improving Fitness

On land, the recommendation for improving fitness is the participation in a minimum of 4-5 aerobic workouts per week. It is further advised that beginning exercisers start their program with 3 exercise sessions per week until they are accustomed to the program.

Due to buoyancy, it is simple to regulate the intensity of the workout in water by either reducing the movement speed, making the movement smaller or allowing buoyancy to support the body for a rest. These variations can sometimes be made while still continuing the movements with the class. Most movements are performed with less impact to the joints and skeletal system and in a cooler environment than land workouts, which may reduce fatigue created by overheating.

Beginning exercisers may adjust comfortably to their water exercise program by applying skills to regulate intensity. Thus, they may be able to increase their frequency and duration of exercise more quickly than with land exercise.

2. Maintaining Fitness (Refer to I. C., Frequency of Aerobic Training, "Basic Exercise Standards and Guidelines").

Maintaining fitness is accomplished by a minimum of 3 workouts evenly spaced throughout the week. Detraining occurs within 2 1/2 weeks or less following cessation of exercise depending on the level and/or fitness level at the time of exercise cessation.

3. Overtraining (Refer to I.C., Frequency of Aerobic Training, "Basic Exercise Standards and Guidelines").

The body needs time to rest, recover and rebuild from the stress of vigorous exercise. Instructors and students should be aware of the symptoms of overtraining that apply the same to land and water exercise (Refer to "Basic Exercise Standards and Guidelines," I.C.3). Additionally, water exercisers should monitor their skin and add extra lotion or Vaseline while the skin is still wet (after a shower) to keep it healthy if necessary. Canvas shoes or aqua socks are recommended for shallow-water workouts to help prevent chafing and slippage.

4. Teaching Fitness

The same guidelines for land instructors apply to water instructors. Water instructors may do all or most of their teaching from the pool deck, and are working with gravity. It is important to note deck instructors should always wear shoes, work safely using low-impact moves and take special care to prevent dehydration by drinking water and cooling off occasionally with a dip in the pool. High air temperatures and humidity make deck teaching difficult. When microphones aren't used, voice overuse is a common problem in a hot, humid, noisy environment.

Again instructors should be aware of the symptoms of overtraining as outlined for land exercise. Individual differences in the number of classes per week an instructor can teach without risk of overtraining depends on the following variables:

a. level of fitness

b. amount of time spent on the deck, intensity and the level of demonstration

c. amount of time spent and level of intensity demonstrating in the water

d. support equipment available, such as a microphone

e. pool environment, air temperature, humidity and exposure to the sun

f. pool water condition and its effect on the skin

g. other fitness activities outside of class

Due to the variations in teaching methods, it is difficult to provide set guidelines. The greatest stress on group instructors during water exercise is to the voice, since pool acoustics tend to be poor, noise levels high and microphones not as readily available (compared to land). The degree of voice use as well as the instructor's response to other variables should be used as a gauge to set the number of classes taught.

Twelve classes per week should be the maximum for the experienced instructor. Check for potential voice overuse and fatigue in setting your own guidelines.

D. To maximize your teaching effectiveness while minimizing your personal risk, a variety of teaching methods can be used in water exercise. The following section examines the pros and cons of some teaching methods for water fitness classes. Instructors must choose a technique that is effective, safe and best meets the objectives for the class.

Method 1: Teaching From the Deck

Pros: It's easy to see students and provide feedback.

Students can see moves easily.

It provides quick visual cues with less instructor voice stress.

The instructor can observe students and pace the workout according to their fitness level.

New students tend to learn the skills more quickly with visual and verbal teaching.

Cons: It's difficult to mimic water moves on land safely and effectively.

High air temperature and slippery surfaces can be dangerous.

Tips: Demo moves at "water speed."

Always wear shoes with traction and impact protection.

Adhere to land training guidelines for safety.

Keep all movement low impact.

Coach, lead and cue, but don't do!

Check student's neck alignment and work away from the pool edge if the front line's necks are hyperextended.

Work on training mats if available to reduce impact.

Use aids such as a chair or stool for mimicking suspended moves.

Wear clothing that is professional and comfortable.

It should provide protection outdoors and allow heat to escape indoors.

Don't yell! Use a microphone if possible.

Demonstrate a move. Then use visual cueing to have students "continue the movement" while you coach them along without performing the move yourself. Provide feedback, motivation and visual cues to change the move during the same move in the progression.

Occasionally, cue close to the water's surface to allow students to maintain good neck and head alignment. When they learn the intensity progression, they can be encouraged to look at each other while keeping their neck in neutral alignment. If they have to keep their eyes glued on a deck instructor, their necks may stay hyperextended throughout the workout. Remember to teach safely on deck. It's a water workout, and you're not in the water.

Method 2: In-Water Teaching

Another method you may enjoy is teaching from the water. Remember, your students can't see your submerged body, so you'll have to use exercise descriptions delivered verbally to students along with visual cues for support.

Students must master the moves before you can teach effectively from the water.

Pros: The instructor shares the workout environment with the student. Hands-on teaching can assist people with learning to trust buoyancy and provide one-on-one corrective feedback for skills improvement.

It's a safer, more fun environment for the instructor.

It may be motivating for the student as you workout together.

Cons: It's difficult for the instructor and students to see the lower body.

Verbal teaching becomes more important, and it may be difficult for people to hear and quickly understand the exercise descriptions.

New students may have a difficult time keeping up with "seasoned" students who understand the skills.

Tips: Wear shoes that provide good in-water traction.

Keep your verbal cues concise and audible.

Perform visual cueing signals high enough above the water for everyone to see, and be sure they understand what they mean.

Wear colored tights and position yourself so you can be seen and move through the class providing feedback.

Ask students "where do you feel the work?" to check for proper exercise execution (it's hard for you to see students now, too). Tell students where they should feel the work.

As students become more skilled, this method becomes more effective and will probably be more fun for you. By mirroring a student, you'll feel their intensity level, share their workout experience and give them support by "matching their move." Say to the class "I'm with Molly now." Everyone has permission to work at their own pace.

Method 3: Combination Method

Many instructors combine in-water teaching with on-the-deck demonstrations. It is a good balance for instructor comfort, safety and fun. But transferring from the deck is difficult. Measure the pros and cons for each of the methods previously discussed and dovetail the best from each technique. The more skills your students understand, the more flexibile the instructor will have to be in the water with them.

Tips: Wear shoes that provide impact protection and have good traction when wet.

Be sure to use safe entrances and exits during transitions.

If your back is turned, be sure the lifeguard is alert.

Deck teach advanced or new skills.

Before you begin a transition, cue students to "continue the move," so they don't stop working.

Give yourself time to adjust to gravity before you begin your deck demonstrations.

Give yourself time to adjust to buoyancy when you reenter the pool.

Plan in advance the deck moves you'll demonstrate, but be flexible enough to ask students during class, "Do you understand the move?"

If you have new students, you may need to deck demo more than water teach until they master the basic skills and understand your cues.

Ask students if they understand the movement during your water lead.

Wear clothing that provides comfort when wet outside of the water and presents a professional appearance without a lot of readjustment during transitions.

Additional Idea: Pre-Class Skills/Class Demonstrations

This technique is recommended to teach new students basic skills they'll need to master for effective water exercise. With students on the pool deck and the instructor in the pool, the instructor can demonstrate and explain the skills. Students get a deck view of the actual skill performed in water and will be better prepared to perform the skill when cued. Allow them to ask questions.

Motivation: Motivation and proper skills performance in water are critical to achieving intensity levels sufficient to elicit training adaptations. Unlike land, a person who simply mimics movements in water without applying force may be working at a lower intensity than required. On land, when everyone lifts their knees up, they all lift against a given load provided by gravity. In water, the force with which a person lifts their knee will determine the load provided by resistance and the amount of buoyancy assisting the leg upwards. On land the leg drops back to the floor effortlessly, while in water, depending on the buoyancy of the leg, the person pushes the leg back into position. That force in water needs to be personally initiated to avoid cheating.

Wide variations in VO_2 responses were demonstrated in two studies (Bishop,1989; Green, 1990) which speculate that the results were due to higher motivation, enthusiasm and higher skill level of some of the subjects. The results imply teaching and motivation techniques used by the exercise leader may affect training results.

Conclusion: Choose a safe teaching style that works for you and your group. Education and skill development will empower students with information so they can take charge of their own workouts and you can enjoy being their coach.

E. Muscle Balancing. (Refer to I.D., Muscle Balancing, "Basic Exercise Standards and Guidelines").

　1. The same principles for muscular balance that apply on land also apply to training in water.

　　In water, the resistance is multi-dimensional providing the opportunity for both the upper and lower body to work in many planes. The arms and legs each have different buoyancies based on body composition and lever length, and must be considered during muscle conditioning exercises. If the arm is "positively buoyant" or "floats," buoyancy will assist movement upward and provide some resistance to movements downward (Fawcett, 1992). For example, during elbow flexion/extension, commonly called a biceps curl exercise, the type of work changes in water and with the equipment used. Let's examine some differences.

When the move is performed on land while holding a dumbbell, the following muscular response occurs:

Biceps: Concentric contraction during elbow flexion
            Eccentric contraction during elbow extension

The same movement performed in water holding a foam dumbbell produces the following response:

Triceps: Eccentric contraction during elbow flexion while resisting buoyancy Concentric contraction during elbow extension

The same movement targets a completely different muscle group in water. If, instead of a foam dumbbell, webbed gloves are worn in the water during the same move, the work changes again.

Biceps: Concentric contraction during elbow flexion

Triceps: Concentric contraction during elbow extension

Instructors must analyze the water's effect on movements to determine what muscle group is being used and how. Intensity for water movements relates to resisting against buoyancy (with foam dumbbells) or applying a combination of surface area and speed (with webbed gloves) to the movement for overload. To achieve maximal speed during the full range of motion, the curl movement should begin at the surface of the water for maximum range of motion for developing speed (by applying more force) in order to maximize intensity. On land, when a weight is picked up, weight is added immediately. In water, overload must be created through range of motion, speed and surface area or buoyancy.

2. Muscle Balancing and Posture

    The training adaptations for water exercise are the same as they are for land. In addition, water provides the opportunity for "on- demand" variable resistance in most planes of movement. The water also is constantly pushing and pulling on the body, and students must be coached to correct trunk alignment for balance. In order to maintain a stabilized torso, to achieve a balanced posture and avoid the risk of low back syndrome, muscles must be balanced in both strength and flexibility. In water, some of the applications are as follows.

    a. Trunk strengthening for the abdominals and erector spinae can be accomplished by performing vertical "abdominal compressions" or stabilization against the resistance of water moving against the body.

Application: During water work, balance is accomplished by contracting abdominals and erector spinae to counteract the forces of moving water against the body. This continuous work in many planes has been shown to produce significant gains in abdominal muscular endurance (Sanders, 1993). Cue students to tuck the hips slightly under to protect the back during travel backwards against resistance, and hold abdominals tight during travel forward to resist against the force pushing the hips backwards. These muscular contractions will train the abdominals using constant vertical compression work, instead of the usual land "crunches." Instructors must cue to constantly remind students to maintain correct posture so they don't relax and allow water to float the hips into hyperextension. Both the abdominals and erector spinae are conditioned during travel moves, providing muscle balance.

b. Back and hamstring flexibility in water can be improved by "yielding" to buoyancy, trusting it to support larger movements (without fear of falling down) than possible to perform on land.

c. The Iliopsoas can be lengthened and released during water exercise by working leg movements to the back of the body. These are easier to balance in water. Specific stretches can also address this area.

d. Proper body alignment will contribute to more effective exercise performance while enhancing abdominal/erector spinae muscular conditioning.

e. For functional muscle balance, Kennedy (1994) recommends the following.

Strengthen:

Shins
Hamstrings
Abdominals
Low Back (Erector Spinae)
Rhomboids & trapezius
Triceps
Inner Thigh Adductors
Latissimus Dorsi

Stretch:

Calves
Quadriceps
Chest (Pectorals)
Hamstrings
Neck
Deltoids
Iliopsoas

f. Balance and posture in water **must** be constantly cued because water acts against the body differently with each exercise.

g. To maintain vertical alignment, muscle isolation occurs during stabilization against the forces surrounding the body.

h. Hyperextension of the knee may occur when the knee and hip are extended during a pull down move from the surface to the pool bottom. Slightly flex the knee to avoid the effect of water's resistance upward against a locked knee.

i. Arching the back in water may occur when the hips are allowed to float backwards, especially during travel forward. If the student has a high amount of body fat on the hips, this may be a natural tendency. It may help to cue for hips under and tight abdominals in order to protect the back and maintain neutral alignment.

j. Both the back and upper body are important for effective posture. Resistance training for these areas by moving the arms and trunk through the water has been shown to be effective. Be sure to use water-specific movements that maximize the water and movement for optimal and "purposeful" (Kennedy, 1994) training.

   k. In order to achieve muscle and joint balance, movements must be worked around the body and joints. Due to the high resistance of water, it is advisable to alternate joint use during sequential muscle overload training. For example, if the biceps muscle has been worked, load resistance on the wrist joint next instead of working the opposing triceps group, which also stresses the elbow. Or, choose a group like the pectorals that requires primary work by the shoulder joint. Sequence muscle balance with regard to joint use and alternate to allow some rest. Remember, however, to work all the muscle group pairs.

E. Body Alignment

The same principles for land apply to water, however, since water buoys the body upwards, allowing larger movements, alignment is more dynamic. Keep these tips in mind for water body alignment and balance.

1. Work the arms and legs in opposition. As the legs are kicking backwards, push your hands through the water forward to balance the lever.

2. Use your hands always to create a "stable base of support." Due to action/reaction, as you push downward through the water the body is assisted upwards. By using your hands on the surface of the water, pressing downward and "sculling," the upper body is supported so your base now includes at least one foot and two hands in shallow water. In deep water or "suspended" in shallow water, the hands can provide enough support to maintain vertical position with the head above the water.

Tuck the navel in and pull it up to cue contraction of the abdorninals during all movements.

During rocking motions backward, place the hands behind you for balance and control as you rock back and keep one leg forward to control the work of the erector spinae and assist with recovery forward. Limit motion backward during rocking moves to a comfortable range as defined by each student.

F. Speed, Isolation and Resistance

The following section addresses water workouts, including resistance and the components of water depth, water temperature, speed and surface area, time, travel and buoyancy which affect resistance levels and intensity progression which applies the components of resistance to water exercises.

1. Resistance

   a. Water Depth

   Before you begin the workout, have students find an effective working depth.

   In shallow water, Kennedy (1989) notes participants exercising in bare feet have a difficult time overcoming inertia to develop speed when they are exercising in nipple-deep water, and heart rates are lower when compared to waist depth.

There is evidence suggesting students must be able to control their movements during shallow water exercise without buoyancy negating their efforts to develop speed. Navel to nipple deep is recommended for most people. If students are too deep, the work will seem easy. If a person is too shallow, the impact is increased. Finding an individual depth to balance gravity and buoyancy allows exercisers to use appropriate speed to control intensity through the water. Deep water exercises are designed differently than shallow water exercises, and control over buoyancy depends on the type and application of buoyancy gear.

b. Water Temperature

There is a neutral temperature at which metabolic heat generated by exercise can be transferred to water without creating an energy cost due to shivering (Cole et al., in press). Maintenance of this thermal balance is important for maximizing optimal training. Exercising with a cool core body temperature can decrease oxygen transport and affect muscular coordination, cardiovascular adjustments and blood flow, intensity and exercise performance (Cole et al., in press; Pendergast, 1988; Craig et al., 1969; Avellini et al., 1983; Svendenhag, 1992). Craig and Dvorak (1968) suggest a neutral temperature (at which heat loss equals heat production for vigorous vertical exercise). In shallow water this would be about 29 C (84 F). To maintain comfort and optimize conditioning, students should be encouraged to keep moving continuously and wear extra clothing. It is recommended facilities maintain a water temperature of around 28-29C (82-84F).

c. Speed

Water provides accommodating resistance to work due to viscosity (Fawcett, 1992). By increasing the speed of movements through the water, drag increases and the muscular force will increase (Cole et al., in press). Unlike on land, the participant also has the force of water acting against the body as well as the force necessary to move the body through the "liquid weight" of water. Evans et al. (1978) found that for walking and jogging in waist deep water, approximately one-half to one-third the speed of land walking/jogging was needed to equal the same level of energy expenditure. This is due to the muscular force required to move through water. Instructors used to teaching at land speed must slow down to accommodate the water.

d. Speed and Surface Area

Speed cannot be considered without regard to surface area moving through the water. Costill (1971) showed work intensities in water are affected proportionately by the surface area moving and the speed of that action determined by the level of muscular strength.

e. Time

Biomechanical analysis of movements, videotaped underwater indicate it takes about four repetitions of a single movement to achieve balance, coordination and maximize range of motion (Sanders & Feroah, 1993). It is recommended that a single move be manipulated through a series of variations that will progressively affect intensity by incorporating the properties of water.

f. Travel

Travel in water creates frontal resistance and form drag and creates greater resistance to movement, thereby increasing the intensity of work (Duffield, 1976). A number of studies indicate oxygen consumption is highest in water when subjects travel though it (Beasley, 1989; Town et al., 1991; Gleim and Nicholas, 1989).

g. Buoyancy

If buoyancy is added for intensity variations, the instructor must examine the direction of resistance against buoyancy, assisting movements upwards, the length of the lever (arms or legs) and speed of movement. Buoyancy gear may also change the shape of the limb or body moving through water, creating some form drag which may increase resistance. However, if speed is slow, this effect may be minimal. Each exercise must be evaluated for the effect of buoyancy on the body and its effect on intensity. Be sure the water depth provides the opportunity for full range of motion below the surface.

2. The Intensity Progression provides the application of the properties for regulating resistance levels.

In water, intensity is regulated by manipulating resistance and buoyancy to create work and rest. In order to regulate resistance on the body, the following Intensity Progression applies the principles of speed, surface area and travel.

The Resistance Intensity Progression

To Increase	To Decrease
Low	High
Increase speed	Stop traveling
Increase surface	Slow Down
(enlarge the move,	Decrease surface
increase range of motion)	(make move smaller,
Increase the speed more	decrease range of motion)
Travel the move	Slow Down more
Increase speed of travel	
High	Low

G. Full Range of Motion

The land principles apply to water also during muscular endurance/strength work. However, since range of motion is used to manipulate overall intensity, it may be necessary to decrease the range of some moves during cardiovascular conditioning to stay within a target range and be able to continue the work. Research has shown there may be a relationship between a minimum level of muscular endurance and the ability to achieve cardiovascular improvements (Sanders, 1993). Due to the high viscosity of water, students may need to target muscular endurance in order to maintain appropriate intensity for a long enough duration to achieve cardiovascular gains. People who are highly conditioned in cardiovascular fitness may need to develop greater muscular endurance to overload in water for additional aerobic conditioning (Kennedy, 1994).

II. Class Format

This is a guideline to class design and format that is physiologically sound and effective and can be adapted to fit most club policies or your personal preference. The following is a recommended sequence for approximately a 1 hour class.

A. Shallow Water

1. Pre-class instruction and equipment orientation

2. Warm-up: (3-5 min.)
   Purpose: To provide a balanced combination of rhythmic limbering exercises, active stretching, water adjustment skills including sculling and recovery to a stand. Easy, continuous movements should be vigorous enough to produce heat for warmth and thermal regulation. Pace the warm-up according to the pool temperature. Instructors should check proper water depth and direct rehearsal of some balanced basic moves that will be used during the workout.

3. Cardio warm-up: (2-3 min.)
   Purpose: To practice traveling moves using proper body alignment and adjustment at a lower intensity, practice sculling to assist propulsion and continue to increase core body temperature and slightly raise heart rate.

4. The Conditioning Phase: (20-40 min.)
   Purpose: To target training to meet fitness goals. It is important to remember to keep the body moving for optimal training. Workouts can be targeted for cardiovascular endurance, muscular strength/endurance or a combination.

B. Guidelines for Targeting Muscle Conditioning

1. Primary Groups: Perform 8-25 repetitions, or until targeted muscles begin to fatigue.

2. Active Rest: Easy jog and scull, 15-30 seconds

   Repeat the sequence: 1-5 sets

3. Intensity: Work at the highest personal level in the Intensity Progression at "Moderate" to "Somewhat Hard." Actively rest and repeat the sequence as needed.

4. Monitor Intensity: Perceived Exertion for muscular fatigue.

5. Assisting Muscle Groups: Enhance overload by providing speed, and contribute to thermal regulation.

6. Alternate joints being "loaded" to reduce stress. If the biceps are targeted, loading the elbow joint, the next upper-body group should target a group such as the pectorals, which loads the shoulder joint.

C. Guidelines for Targeting the Workout for Cardiovascular Endurance

1.	Duration:	Perform continuous movements for a 5-8 minute cardiovascular set. Link sets to comply with ACSM guidelines.
2.	Intensity:	Maintain an intensity level that allows you to perform continuous exercise, coordinating both arm and leg work for aerobic conditioning according to the ACSM guidelines. Focus on lower body work for cardiovascular fitness, and before you become breathless, lower the intensity by manipulating moves in the Intensity Progression. Change to a new move before the working muscles fatigue.
3.	Active Rest:	Continue the movement at the lower end of the progression or perform a resting jog/scull.
4.	Monitor Intensity:	"Talk Test," or a combination of the "Talk Test and Heart Rate" or Perceived Exertion.

D. The Intensity Progressions

1. Upper body applications

Only use webbed gloves or hands for support, slicing and webbing softly for balance. Aerobic conditioning depends on the lower body creating the work. When the arms are added, heart rate may elevate artificially.

2. Lower body applications

Perform a sequence of moves using the Intensity Progression. To maintain intensity, vary movements before muscles become fatigued but allow enough time for students to balance and develop a movement so water can act against the body to create training.

E. Equipment Application for Overload in the Progression

Various equipment designed for water exercise can further amplify the effect of water's resistance on the body. Basically, equipment falls into one of the following categories.

1. Buoyancy enhancement.

2. Surface area enhancement.

3. A combination of buoyancy and surface area adjustment.

Instructors must evaluate the purpose for each piece, design movements based on the properties of water and principles of exercise science and evaluate each for function and safety before adding it to the program. Each piece of equipment will have its own program or movement types. Some common gear for "overload" includes:

1. Buoyancy: foam dumbbells, belts or tubes.

2. Surface area: webbed gloves, fins

3. Combination: "sloggers" (giant sandals), foam cuffs worn on the ankles.

   The aquatic step used during shallow water workouts affects intensity by allowing students to increase range of motion and speed and providing a small shallow water area that allows students to add more gravity into the work on the step while providing the safe cushion of the deeper water for recovery off the step.

F. **Cool-down: (2-3 min.)**

   Purpose: To promote gradual reduction in cardiovascular function while maintaining body warmth with light, easy buoyant movements.

G. **Active Stretching and Warm Down: (3-6 min.)**

   Purpose: To increase range of motion, relax and exit the pool feeling warm. Stretching may be performed here if the water temperature allows without significant body cooling. By sculling with the upper body during lower body work, and jogging during upper body work, you can help maintain body warmth. The warm down provides easy, light buoyant movements which allow the body to warm back up, so students leave the pool without feeling chilled.

H. **Deep Water**

   1. Equipment orientation and safety skills check
      Purpose: To check deep water comfort and safety skills, and teach equipment application. Students should be comfortable in deep water, be able to perform recovery to a vertical position and be able to tread water or "swim" their way to the side of the pool before being allowed to go into the deep end, even with equipment on.

   2. Warm-up: (3-5 min.)
      Purpose: To learn adjustment and balance with equipment, to learn buoyancy and to adjust to water temperature.

   3. Stabilization and sculling: (3-5 min.)
      Purpose: To practice trunk alignment in various body positions and assist balance using sculling skills.

   4. Cardio warm-up: (2-3 min.)
      Purpose: For students to practice body alignment and locomotion methods during travel moves.

   5. Conditioning sets targeting either cardiovascular endurance or muscular strengthening and endurance.

   6. Endurance Conditioning: (20-40 min.)
      Purpose: To target training for specific fitness goals.

   7. Active stretch and warm down: (3-8 min.)
      Purpose: Same as shallow water.

8. Transition to shallow water (if possible) and perform easy, shallow water moves, without buoyancy or resistance gear for 2-3 min.
Purpose: To prepare students for gravity and decrease intensity further.

III. Class Level

Since each person varies with regard to body composition, fat deposition, skill and fitness level, response to water is individual. Coach to allow students to work at their own pace by teaching them the Intensity Progression and encouraging them to adjust the components to match their own body composition, skills and fitness level. Since intensity is regulated in water by using speed, it is not advised to encourage students to work either on the beat of the music or to your counting. Individualize the workouts by teaching skills and giving feedback for motivation and improvement without driving the pace. Music can be used to provide an atmosphere of fun and encouragement, but must not dictate movement speed.

IV. Instructional Methods, Concerns and Responsibility

A. Monitoring
Purpose:

1. Maximizing exercise effectiveness

2. Injury prevention

The same guidelines listed for land apply in water, with the following additions.

Panic—wide eyes, stiffness, obvious fear of water
Body Core Cooling—shivering, blue lips, pinched face and hands folded over the chest to stay warm.

B. Cueing

All of the same principles from land apply to the water with some additional considerations. Water instructors leading from the deck must not try to participate in the exercises. It is impossible to perform a water workout perfectly on the deck, and the instructor should focus on teaching students instead of getting a personal workout.

Allow time for the student to practice or "mark" the move. Then, coach them through the intensity progression and watch carefully to provide corrective feedback. To protect your voice, use hand signals if you don't have a microphone.

V. Legal Responsibilities

Legal responsibilities are the same as those for land with the following amendments.

A. Water Fitness instructors should complete training that tests both theoretical knowledge and performance skills for the application of land-based exercise methods to the water environment, combining the sciences of exercise and water.

B. Water Fitness instructors should have a basic knowledge about Emergency Water Safety Skills and be able to assist with the response in the event of a water emergency.

C. A lifeguard should be on duty during classes. If this is not possible, the Water Fitness instructor must be **currently** certified in Lifeguard Training, CPR and have an Emergency Action Plan developed for each facility.

D. The facility must provide basic safety equipment along with a safe environment, including balanced water chemicals, clear water, a clean facility and safe water temperature.

VI. Pre-Class Procedures

A. Medical Clearance

All the land-based items apply with the following additions (Refer to "Basic Exercise Standards and Guidelines," IV.A.). Individuals should not be encouraged to participate in water exercise if they have diminished respiratory functions or capacity, suffer from bladder or vaginal infections or have been diagnosed with severe hypotension. Additionally, individuals who suffer from known allergies, have an infectious disease or who have post-surgery open wounds (including a recent episiotomy) should be discouraged from participating in water exercise. Check with your local facility or Health Department for additional medical restrictions in your area.

Finally, a person who is afraid of water will not relax enough to enjoy and benefit from a water exercise program. Panic is a leading cause of drowning, and it can occur even in shallow water. People who are afraid of water but are interested in a water exercise program should be encouraged to take a basic learn-to-swim course in order to develop water adjustment skills prior to a water fitness program.

B. Facility Check and Introductions

Before class it is the responsibility of the instructor to scan the pool and deck area for hazards such as broken glass, debris, broken ladders or slippery areas. Dangerous situations, however minor, must be corrected or pointed out to students. Check the pool and deck before each class. Check the water temperature and set up your music system away from the water's edge. If your students shower before entering the pool, you must begin managing their thermal regulation immediately to prevent body chilling, so organization and attention to their movements are imperative.

C. Attire

Shoes should be worn to increase traction, for safety and for cleanliness. Instructors should wear tights or suits that provide adequate coverage when a student looks up from the pool to you on the deck, and when you are getting in and out of the pool for demonstrations. A professional appearance provides more focus on learning.

D. Level of Participation

Check to be sure everyone is comfortable in water and can recover to a stand if they lose their balance. Teach the intensity progression, sculling and explain how to monitor intensity using perceived exertion and the "talk test." Explain that they must keep moving continuously to stay warm. Show them proper entrances and identify the working area and depths. The recommendations for land-based exercise apply also.

E. Breathing

The same basic breathing principles apply for water (Refer to "Basic Exercise Standards and Guidelines," IV.E.). Encourage breathing especially during "suspended" or deep water exercise. When hydrostatic pressure of water pushes against the lungs, some students will "top breathe," or perform shallow breaths, since it feels more difficult to inflate the lungs against pressure. Cue them to breathe.

F. Orientation to Water

Provide some brief tips on feeling buoyancy, finding a working depth, good postural alignment in water and monitoring intensity. Point out some differences between land and water and how much different the exercises will feel (cooler, lighter, speed varies the work). Simply using land-based movements in water may not optimize training. The properties of buoyancy, and resistance created by surface area, speed and movement through water need to be taught. Advise them that buoyancy will make them want to dance on their toes and encourage them to practice pressing their heels to the bottom occasionally to avoid calf cramps, a common complaint from beginners.

VII. Water-Specific Items that Address Workout Components

A. Special Considerations for Prenatal.

Prenatal—The American College of Obstetricians and Gynecologists (ACOG) has recently revised their recommendations for exercise prescriptions during pregnancy. Use these guidelines to coach students who are pregnant and attending your program. A few tips to remember for your water fitness prenatal students include:

1. ACOG guidelines (1994) state "women can continue to exercise and derive health benefits even from mild-to-moderate exercise routines" (ACOG Technical Bulletin, Number 189-February, 1994, page 3).

2. Cool water exercise may help regulate maternal core temperature. However, exercise in warm water should be avoided.

3. Avoid cold water and/or airflow which may stimulate nipple erection and hormone changes.

4. Wear supportive swimwear and jog bra for protection from chafing.

5. Protect softened connective tissue affected by relaxin by promoting muscle strength.

6. Limit the range of motion during hip extension/flexion moves to avoid stress on the broad and/or round ligament.

7. Limit rebound moves and quick changes in direction.

8. Reinforce proper body alignment.

9. Vary the muscle groups to balance blood shunting and avoid fatigue.

10. Encourage hydration before, during and after exercise bouts.

B. Questionable Exercises for the General Population

Exercises that should be considered for potential risk for the general population:

1. Double leg raises while hanging backwards on the pool wall. This exercise creates excessive pressure on the lumbar disks (Thomas & Rippee, 1992).

2. One leg on pool gutter with forward flexion for a hamstring stretch may overload the lumbar spine and does not effectively stretch the targeted muscle. This exercise may also cause piroformis syndrome (Corbin & Lindsey, 1994).

3. Full "crunches" with legs hooked over the pool gutter.

4. Crossing legs midline of the body if there has been a hip replacement.

5. Avoid full leg extensions after ACL knee surgery.

6. Decrease forward speed and stabilize the spine during travel moves with students suffering from back problems.

7. For students with a history of shoulder dislocation, limit shoulder external rotation to 20 degrees back, behind the body.

8. Lifting weighted objects like jugs filled with water overhead while the body is partially submerged compromises balance, could impinge the shoulder joint and dramatically increases blood pressure.

9. Repetitive arm work above the surface of the water stresses the shoulder joint and does not contribute significantly to aerobic conditioning. Research tells us that arm cranking moves as well as arm work above the head produce a higher heart rate relative to VO_2 demands (Shepard, 1984; Astrand,1968). Resistive work with the arms produces relatively low oxygen uptake and does not meet the criteria for aerobic training intensity (Beasely, 1989) due to the presser response. Above water arm work should be limited and functional.

10. Adding land weights to a water workout should be limited to physical therapy work only. There are many risks to be considered with this method of overload.

11. Full push-ups upwards using the wall or gutter should be evaluated for individual safety and performance. (Refer to "Basic Exercise Standards & Guidelines," VIII. F.)

Evaluate the cost and benefits of each exercise. Any movement that compromises good body alignment should be reevaluated. Remember to determine the direction of buoyancy and resistance acting against the body and examine the resulting contractions needed to maintain alignment. If an exercise can be done differently and more safely, modify it.

C. Monitoring Intensity in Water

Heart rates are difficult to assess accurately, even during land exercise (Ebbeling et al, 1991). In water, assessing heart rate is even more difficult and seems to be less effective due to a wide number of variables such as motivation, fitness level, water temperature, clothing worn by the student, water depth and exercise types (McArdle, et al., 1976; Ritchie & Hopkins, 1991). Navia (1986) and Ritchie & Hopkins (1991) suggest lower heart rates in water may correlate with an aerobic training effect on land expected from a higher heart rate. Because of the inconclusive evidence and seeming contradictions, it is recommended that participants use a combination of perceived exertion, the "Talk Test" and heart rates (if they are highly skilled) to determine exercise intensity.

D. Music

1. Choose music that's fun and motivating. It's suggested you use a variety of tempos, sounds and styles to give a sense of excitement and energy. Remember it takes individual effort to press through the resistance of water, and music can motivate. However, since intensity is regulated by speed, allow students to work on their own beat, not yours or the music's.

2. During muscular conditioning sets, you may want to use a continuous type tape with a pace about 120-130 beats per minute to provide motivation and variety. The duration of the repetitions and sets can be changed according to the group's fitness level, not song length, and the beat is energetic enough to motivate.

3. For aerobic conditioning classes, various 3-8 minute songs provide opportunities to change the type and mood of continuous exercise.

4. It is extremely difficult to provide safe and effective training for everyone while working to the music beat. Allow students to enjoy the music, working at their own intensity and beat (pace). Different body types react differently in water, and the student's own force and speed provide a personal level of resistance for self-directed training.

E. Saunas and Hot Tubs

Saunas, hot tubs and hot showers may be appropriate after water exercise when the body has chilled. Encourage students to warm up if they feel chilled. Average pool water temperature and a wet body in cool air will make the body feel cool as the workout begins to slow down. Overheating the body should be avoided, so limit exposure after exercise.

F. Hydration

The principles of hydration apply the same in water as they do on land. Sometimes people think because they are exercising in water, they don't need to drink water. Also, since heat stress is not as much of a problem in water, thirst may not be stimulated in the same way it is during land classes. Moisture is lost through sweat and respiration, and as these factors increase during water exercise, the body must be hydrated to avoid fatigue. Have students bring water bottles and encourage them to drink periodically.

G. Exercise Design Considerations

1. Students must be taught how to use their hands to coordinate every move in water and provide a stable base of support. For the most effective training, hands should be used primarily in the water to optimize the resistance and support it provides. Webbed gloves are highly recommended to provide a larger surface area that encourages a slower speed of the hand through water and more effectively matches the slower speed of the lower body. Coordinating the larger, more buoyant moves will be easier when upper and lower body speeds are more closely matched. Additionally, webbed gloves provide more efficient sculling motions to assist with travel and balance and offer a progressive overload for upper body training.

2. Shoes should be worn during all shallow water workouts to provide traction for maximal speed and protection.

3. Land-based movements do not necessarily optimize water training. Two training studies (Simpson, 1994; Abraham, 1994) which used land based moves, one on the Aquatic Step and the other during a rhythmic shallow water program, show no significant improvements in cardiovascular endurance. This contradicts results from other studies which report significant gains in cardiovascular conditioning with land-based moves (Barretta, 1994; Hoeger, 1993; Sanders, 1993; Ruoti, 1994). These programs may have addressed the properties of water with their exercise design more effectively. Optimization of water for training results requires you to modify land movements for water and apply intensity progressions to provide individualized water-specific work.

4. Abdominals are trained in a functional vertical stance in water. Research by Sanders (1993) supports vertical abdominal compression during dynamic postural alignment against the water's buoyancy and resistance to train the trunk muscles. This technique should be used constantly during class, so abdominal isolation work is not needed. Cue students to proper alignment and give corrective feedback for improvements.

References

American College of Sports Medicine (1991). The recommended quantity and quality of exercise for developing and maintaining cardiorespiratory and muscular fitness in healthy adults. *The official position papers of the american college of sports medicine* (6th ed.), or *Medicine and Science in Sports and Exercise*, 22: 2 (1990): 265-74.

American Council on Exercise (1993). *Aerobics instructor manual*. Variations Chapter. Ca.: ACE.

Astrand, I., Guharay, A., & Wahren, J. (1968). Circulatory responses to arm exercise with different arm positions. *Journal of Applied Physiology*, 25: 528-32.

Avellini, B., Shapiro, Y., & Pandolf, K. (1983). Cardiorespiratory physical training in water and on land. *European Journal of Applied Physiology and Occupational Physiology*, 53: 255-63.

Barretta, R. (1993). Physiological training adaptations to a 14-week, deep water exercise program. Unpublished dissertation, University of New Mexico, Albuquerque.

Beasley, B. (1989). Prescription pointers on aquatic exercise. *Sports Medicine Digest*, 11:1.

Brennan, D.K., Michaud, T.J., Wilder, R.P., & Sherman, N.W. (1992). Gains in aquarunning peak oxygen consumption after eight weeks of aquarun training. *Medicine and Science in Sports and Exercise*, 24: 5: S23.

Cassady, S.L., & Nielsen, D.H. (1992). Cardioirespiratory responses of healthy subjects to calisthenics performed on land versus in water. *Physical Therapy*, 72:7: 62/532-68/538.

Cole, A., Moschetti,; M., & Eagleston, R.E. (in press). Lumbar spine aquatic rehabilitation. In A. Cole (Ed.), *A sports medicine approach, Handbook of pain management* (2nd ed.). Baltimore: Williams & Wilkins.

Corbin, C.B., & Lindsey, R. (1994). *Concepts of physical fitness* (8th ed.). Madison, Wi.: Brown & Benchmark.

Costill, D.L. (1971). Energy requirements during exercise in the water. *Journal of Sports Medicine*, 11: 87-92.

Costill, D., Cahill, P.J., & Eddy, D. (1967). Metabolic responses to submaximal exercise in three water temperatures. *Journal of Applied Physiology*: 22: 628-32.

Craig, A., & Dvorak, M. (1969). Comparison of exercise in air and in water of different temperatures. *Medicine and Science in Sports and Exercise*, 1:3: 124-30.

Craig, A.B., Jr., & Dvorak, M. (1968). Thermalregulation of man during water of different temperatures. *Journal of Applied Physiology*: 25: 23-35.

Duffield, M.H. (1976). *Exercise in water*. Baltimore: Williams & Wilkins.

Ebbeling, C.B., Ebbeling, C.J., Ward, A., & Rippe, J. (1991). Comparison between palpated heart rates and the heart rates observed using the polar favor heart rate monitor during aerobics exercise class. (Unpublished study). Exercise Physiology and Nutrition Laboratory, University of Massachusetts Medical School.

Eckerson, J., & Anderson, T. (1992). Physiological response to water aerobics. *The Journal of Sports Medicine and Physical Fitness*, 32: 3: 255-61.

Evans, B.W., Cureton, K.J., & Purvis, J.W. (1978). Metabolic and circulatory responses to walking and jogging in water. *Research Quarterly*, 49: 442-49.

Fawcett, C.W. (Summer, 1992). Principles of aquatic rehab: A new look at hydrotherapy. *Sports Medicine*, 7: 2: 6-9).

Fernhall, B., Manfredi, T., & Congdon, K. (1992). Prescribing water-based exercise from treadmill and arm ergometry in cardiac patients. *Medicine and Science in Sports and Exercise*, 24:1: 139-43.

Gleim, G.W., & Nicholas, J.A. (March-April, 1989). Metabolic costs and heart rate responses to treadmill walking in water a different depths and temperatures. *American Journal of Sports Medicine*, 5: 248.

Graham, T.E. (1988). Thermal, metabolic and cardiovascular changes in men and women during cold stress. *Medicine and Science in Sports and Exercise*, 20:5: S185-91.

Gwimup, G. (1987). Weight loss without dietary restriction: Efficacy of different forms fo aerobic exercise. *American Journal of Sports Medicine*, 15:3: 275-79.

Hoeger, W., Gibson, T., Moore, J., & Hopkins, D. (Winter, 1993). A comparison of selected training responses to water aerobics and low impact aerobic dance. *National Aquatics Journal*, 13-16.

Hoeger, W.K., Hopkins, D.R., Barber, D.J., & Gibson,; T. (1992). Comparison of maximal VO2, HR and RPE between treadmill running and water aerobics. *Medicine and Science in Sports and Exercise*, 24:5: S96.

Kennedy, C. (1994). Search for water exercise choices. Paper presented at AEA Conference. Champaign, Ill.: (217) 244-0261.

Kennedy, C., Foster, V., Harris, M., & Stokler, J. (October, 1989). The influence of music tempo and water depth on heart rate response to aqua aerobics. Paper presented at IDEA Foundation International Symposium on the Medical and Scientific Aspects of Aerobic Dance, San Diego, Ca.

Knecht, S. (1992). Physical and psychological changes accompanying a 10-week aquatic exercise program. AKWA Letter, 5:5: 6.

Lowis, S. (1994). *Waterbellies, Aquatic training for the pre/postnatal instructor*. Tahoe City, Ca. 96145.

Maharam, L.G. (1992). Swim yourself thin? *Fitness Swimmer Magazine* (June): 50-51.

McArdle, W.D., Magel, J.R., Lesmes, G.R., & Pechar, G.S. (1976). Metabolic and cardiovascular adjustment to work in air and water at 18°, 25° and 33° C. *Journal of Applied Physiology*, 40: 85-90.

McArdle, W.D., Katch, F.I., & Katch, V.L. (1991). *Exercise physiology, energy, nutrition, and human performance* (3rd ed.). Philadelphia and London: Lea & Febiger.

Michaud, T.J., Brennan, D.K., Wilder, R.P., & Sherman, N.W. (1992). Aquarun training and changes in treadmill running, maximal oxygen consumption. *Medicine and Science in Sports & Exercise*, 24: 5: S23.

Miss, M. (1988). Comparison between the effects of a nine-week exercise program on land or in the water on selected components of pysical fitness. Master's Thesis, The University of Illinios at Chicago.

Navia, A.M. (1986). Comparison of energy expenditure between treadmill running and water running. Thesis, University of Alabama, Birmingham.

Pendergast, D.R. (1988). *Medicine and Science in Sports and Exercise*, 20:5: Supplement, S170-175.

Rennie, D.W. (1988). Tissue heat transfer in water: Lessons from the Korean divers. *Medicine and Science in Sports and Exercise*, 20:5: S177-S183.

Rippee, N., Sanders, M. (1994). Probing the depths of water fitness research. *IDEA Today* (August).

Ritchie, S., & Hopkins, W. (1991). The intensity of deep water running. *International Journal of Sports Medicine*, 12: 27-29.

Ruoti, G., Troup, J., & Berger, R. (1994). The effects of nonswimming water exercises on older adults. *Journal of Sport & Physical Therapy*, 19:3 (March).

Sanders, M., & Feroali, A. (1993). Biomechanical analysis of a water fitness movement using the ariel performance analysis computer system. Unpublished data, Reno Orthopaedic and Sports Medicine Clinic, Reno, Nevada.

Sanders, M., & Rippee, N. (1994). Speedo aquatic exercise instructor training video. Speedo USA/Authentic Fitness Products.

Sanders, M.E. (1992). The art & science of wave aerobics. Video Course. Fitness Wholesale.

Sanders, M.E. (1993). Selected physiological training adaptations during a water fitness program called Wave Aerobics. Thesis, University of Nevada, Reno, Microform Publications, University of Oregon, Eugene.

Sanders, M., Rippee, N. (1994). Speedo's Aquatic Fitness System, Instructor Training Workbook. Speedo International, Ltd., London, England.

Shephard, R. (1984). Tests of maximal oxygen uptake: A critical review. *Sports Medicine*, 7: 77-80.

Simpson, A., & Miller, M. (1994). Aquastep your way to fitness. Unpublished data, University of Wisconsin-La Crosse, Department of Physical Education.

Stavish, J.M. (1987). Walk-jog versus swim training: Effects on body composition and aerobic capacity. Unpublished thesis, San Diego State University, San Diego, California.

Stevenson, J., Tacia, S., Thompson, J., & Crane, C. (1988). A comparison of land and water exercise programs for older individuals. *Medicine and Science in Sports and Exercise*, S537.

Svedenhag, J., & Seger, J., (1992). Running on land and in water: Comparative exercise physiology. *Medicine and Science in Sports and Exercise*, 1155-1160.

Thomas, D.Q., & Long, K.A. (1994). Generalizability of deep water exerciser blood pressure. *Research Quarterly for Exercise and Sport*, 65S (March): A-30.

Thomas, D.Q., & Rippee, N.E. (1993). *Is your aerobics class killing you?* Chicago: Acapella Books.

Town, G.P., & Bradley, S.S. (1991). Maximal metabolic responses of deep and shallow water running in trained runners. *Medicine & Science in Sports & Exercise*, 23:2: 238-241.

Whitley, J.D., & Schoene, L.L. (1987). Comparison of heart rate reponses; Water walking versus treadmill walking. *Physical Therapy*, 67: 1501-1504.

Wilder, R., Brennan, D., & Schottee, D. (1993). A standard measure for exercise prescription for aqua running. *American Journal of Sports Medicine*, 21:1: 45-48.

Wilder, R.P., & Brennan, D.K. (1993). Physiological responses to deep water running in athletes. *Sports Medicine*, 16:6: 374-380.

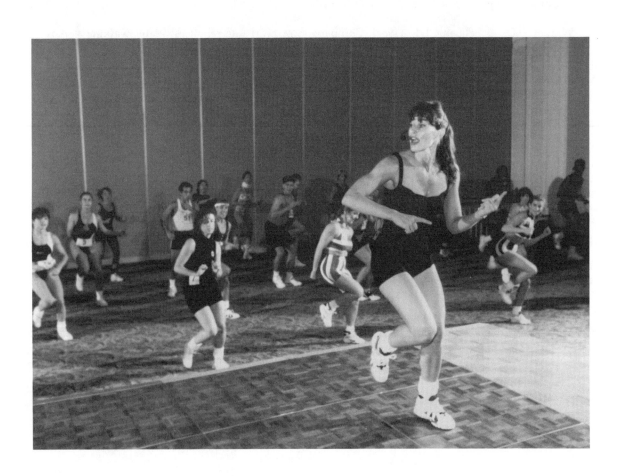

STANDARDS AND GUIDELINES

of the

Aerobics and Fitness Association of America

for

Non-Weighted
Low-Impact Aerobics

I. Basic Principles, Definitions and Recommendations

All Standards and Guidelines outlined as follows apply to average adults without known physiological or medical conditions that would in any way restrict their exercise activities. These Standards and Guidelines are designed to be used in conjunction with "Basic Exercise Standards and Guidelines of the Aerobics and Fitness Association of America."

A. Definitions

Low-impact aerobics is a form of cardiovascular exercise in which each of the movement patterns is performed with one foot in contact with the floor at all times. By keeping one foot on the floor, the amount of stress associated with the impetus of floor contact is significantly lessened. Low-impact does not necessarily imply the class is performed at a low intensity, as the intensity may vary from beginning to advanced levels, depending on exercise selection, exercise sequencing and movement patterns. Low-impact aerobics may be performed with or without hand weights (see "Standards and Guidelines for Weighted Workouts"). Other popular names for low-impact aerobics are: light aerobics, moderate aerobics and controlled-impact.

By contrast, a **high-impact** or **combination** aerobics class contains movements whereby one or both feet can leave the floor, such as jogging, hopping, skipping and jumping.

A **non-impact** class contains no movement patterns such as stepping, walking or leg lifts as both feet remain firmly planted on the floor throughout the exercises being performed. This may include upper torso strengthening, squats or squat lunges in place.

B. Who Should Participate

Low-impact aerobics provides excellent cardiovascular conditioning when performed according to the training principles of frequency, intensity and duration. Many individuals participate in low-impact aerobics as an alternative activity to other more stressful, high-impact exercise modes such as running or high-impact aerobics. Low-impact aerobics is well suited to virtually any healthy individual, if performed safely according to recommended training principles, and ideal for those who must restrict stress to the knees, feet, lower legs and hips. All individuals beginning an exercise program should follow the guidelines for medical clearance as stated in "Basic Exercise Standards and Guidelines," section IV.A.

II. Training Principles and Guidelines

A. Frequency

For aerobic training to occur, low-impact aerobics without weights should be performed 3-5 times per week. As in other forms of cardiovascular conditioning, 3 times a week will maintain current aerobic training levels for the active individual, and 4-5 workouts per week may be necessary to produce improvements, depending upon other training factors and additional weekly activity.

B. Intensity

1. Training Effect

   To provide an aerobic training effect, a non-weighted low-impact class should provide sufficient overload to maintain an individual's heart rate within his/her training heart rate range of 55-85% of estimated maximum heart rate. The aerobic portion should resemble a normal bell curve, as recommended for high-impact aerobics (see "Basic Exercise Standards and Guidelines," section VI.C). Intensity will vary depending on exercise selection, movement patterns and sequencing, elevated movement, speed and lever length. These variables should be utilized according to the fitness level of the class.

2. Exercise Selection

   The variety of movements used and choice of exercise appropriate for an individual's fitness level will be a determining factor in raising or lowering exercise intensity as well as maintaining a consistent intensity level throughout the aerobic portion of the class. Also, choose a variety of exercises that will both utilize and balance the large muscle groups of the body. For example, if you do a lot of knee lifts which use the quadriceps and hip flexors, balance these with hip extensions which use the opposing muscles, the hamstrings and gluteals.

3. Movement Patterns and Sequencing

   Sequence of movement patterns is another controlling factor of intensity in a low-impact workout because the exercises chosen as part of a combination and/or pattern can either increase, decrease or maintain aerobic intensity. In a low-impact class, the intensity can be increased by building a sequence that varies the elevation of arm and leg movements. This can be accomplished with combinations in place or by traveling, utilizing available space and moving across the floor in a continuous pattern. Increase intensity levels through movement patterns as a gradual progression. During a steady state, develop successive combinations that will be of similar intensity levels to maintain heart rate.

4. Elevated Movements

Intensity of an exercise can be influenced by the elevation at which it is performed. Elevating the legs, e.g., a knee lift compared to a heel dig, is a way to increase intensity as more work is being required of the large muscle groups, resulting in increased cardiac output and elevated heart rate. Raising the arms above the head, particularly for an extended period of time will similarly increase heart rate. However, this is a false reading due to the pressor response. Pressor response is when arm movements are performed above the head, elevating heart rate but not increasing cardiac output. Therefore, to accurately increase exercise intensity, vary arm movements between high, middle and low ranges to avoid the pressor response. At the same time, continue to utilize elevated leg movements as the way to increase intensity, using appropriate arm combinations.

5. Speed

Speed of movement during a low-impact class will have a direct effect on increased heart rate. Movement either in place or in traveling patterns across the floor should be performed through a full range of motion with control. Use of speed to move across the floor is appropriate if momentum and alignment are controlled. Maximum movement speed for a non-weighted aerobic workout should be 150 bpm with a recommended range of 116-145 bpm.

6. Lever Length

Arm or leg exercises that use extended levers (e.g., straight arms in a horizontal position as opposed to bent elbows in the same position) will increase the workload or intensity of the movement due to the amount of force required to move the lever (in this case an arm) against gravity. It is also more difficult to control movement without momentum through a full range of motion and maintain proper body alignment with the use of longer levers. Long lever movements should be modified for beginners or interspersed with short lever movements in sequencing patterns as a means of controlling intensity.

C. Duration

For cardiovascular conditioning, a non-weighted low-impact class should include a minimum of 20 minutes and up to 45 minutes of aerobic activity within an individual's training heart rate range. Additional time of 8-12 minutes should be incorporated for an appropriate warm-up period that includes both rhythmic limbering movements and static stretches to facilitate range of motion development and injury prevention (see "Basic Exercise Standards and Guidelines," section V). An additional 2-3 minutes at the end of the aerobic portion should be allotted for an appropriate post-aerobic cool-down to gradually decrease aerobic intensity and heart rate (see "Basic Exercise Standards and Guidelines," section VII).

D. Overload

A training effect will occur when muscles are regularly overloaded beyond the level to which they are accustomed (see "Basic Exercise Standards and Guidelines" section I.B). Overload is accomplished by increasing resistance, repetitions, sets and/or varying intensity with any of the variables listed in section II.B of this chapter.

E. Muscle Strengthening

Muscular strengthening can be achieved in a low-impact class without the use of added weight by the same methods utilized in traditional aerobic and body conditioning classes with non-weighted floorwork (see "Basic Exercise Standards and Guidelines," sections VIII-XI). Factors to control include body position, muscle isolation, range of motion, repetitions and exercise sequence.

F. Posture and Alignment

See "Basic Exercise Standards and Guidelines," section I.E, as well as alignment for specific body positions in sections V and VIII-XI. In addition, be aware of body balance in low-impact positions and movements.

III. Class Format

A. Sequence

The order in which certain exercises are performed is important. For example, a warm-up should precede all other activity (see "Basic Exercise Standards and Guidelines," section II.A-B). The following is the recommended sequence as adapted by AFAA for a one-hour, non-weighted low-impact class:

1. Pre-class Instruction
2. Warm-up should be a balanced combination of rhythmic limbering exercises designed to prepare the body for the stress of more vigorous exercise and static stretching. Follow guidelines recommended for warm-up in "Basic Exercise Standards and Guidelines," section V.
3. Low-impact aerobics for cardiovascular conditioning and post-aerobic cool-down
4. Standing muscular strengthening for upper and/or lower body. (If using weights, see the following chapter, "Standards and Guidelines for Weighted Workouts.")
5. Floorwork, in order of preference:
    a. Legs
    b. Buttocks
    c. Hips
    d. Abdominals
    e. Lower back

(If using weights, see "Standards and Guidelines for Weighted Workouts," sections IX-XIV.)

6. Final static stretch cool-down

IV. Pre-Class Procedure

A. Instructor Checklist

Review points to cover in "Basic Exercise Standards and Guidelines," section IV.

1. Medical clearance
2. Level of participation
3. Appropriate shoes
4. Breathing
5. Aerobics orientation
6. Heart rate monitoring and perceived exertion levels

B. Low-impact Orientation

Familiarize students with important body alignment cues for maintaining proper positioning as well as receiving optimal fitness benefits from a low-impact workout. Review the following important points, using demonstration if necessary:

1. Complete all movements through the full range of motion.
2. Control speed.
3. If possible, use both arms and legs during combinations and moving patterns to maintain workout intensity.
4. Modify any movements to accommodate individual needs.

V. Warm-Up

A. Purpose

Prepares the body for vigorous exercise and may reduce the risk of injury.

B. Time

Class should always begin with an 8-12 minute warm-up, including exercises specific to muscles that will be utilized during the workout.

C. Specific Warm-up Guidelines

The guidelines for static stretching, rhythmic limbering exercises, warm-up sequencing, muscle groups utilized, and special do's and don'ts (as described in "Basic Exercise Standards and Guidelines," section V) should be followed for a non-weighted low-impact class.

VI. Aerobics

A. Time

20-45 minutes is recommended, not including warm-up or post-aerobic cool-down.

B. Sequence

1. Start slowly and gradually increase the intensity and range of motion of your movements. All considerations discussed in "Basic Exercise Standards and Guidelines," section VI, should be adhered to until such time as a steady state has been achieved—approximately 3-5 minutes after the aerobic portion has begun.

2. Low-impact aerobics is characterized by a variety of foot patterns, high stepping or marching and the absence of jogging. One foot remains on the ground at all times. Movements are controlled, utilize full range of motion, are non-ballistic and work best by incorporating creative arm combinations with foot patterns.

3. Heart rate should be maintained in the 55-85% range of estimated maximum heart rate (see "Basic Exercise Standards and Guidelines," section VI.I, for calculation and monitoring methods). Heart rate may be elevated or decreased by regulating the intensity of the exercise. Factors affecting intensity may be found in section II.C of this chapter.

C. Special Considerations

1. When lunging, knees should be aligned directly over the feet; don't overshoot toes or medially rotate the hip so the knee is no longer aligned with the foot.

2. Keep body weight balanced over arches; avoid leaning forward.

3. Avoid repetitive overuse of hip flexor movements; balance exercise selection.

VII. Post-Aerobic Cool-Down

A. Purpose

To provide a transition period between vigorous aerobic work and less taxing exercise, allowing working heart rate to return to pre-exercise rate safely without overstressing cardiovascular functions.

B. Time

2-5 minutes is recommended.

C. Type of Movement

Rhythmic movement that gradually decreases in speed and range of motion.

D. Method

Use moderate to slow rhythmic movements for both upper and lower body, followed by static stretches for the upper back, shoulders, arms as well as calves, quadriceps, hamstrings, front of shins and lower back. Pay particular attention to muscles utilized in the aerobic portion. Check heart rate. Heart rate should be at 60% or less of the working heart rate before beginning any floorwork. Either conclude with static stretches, if the class is a cardiovascular workout only, or proceed to any strengthening activities listed in section III.A of this chapter.

VIII. Strengthening Exercises for Upper and Lower Body

A. Strengthening Without the Use of Weights

If strengthening exercises without weights are to be included for upper (arms, chest, shoulders and upper back) and/or lower body (legs, hips, buttocks, abdominals and lower back), see "Basic Exercise Standards and Guidelines," sections VIII-XI.

B. Strengthening With the Use of Weights

If strengthening exercises with weights are to be included for either upper or lower body, see "Standards and Guidelines for Weighted Workouts," sections VIII-XIV.

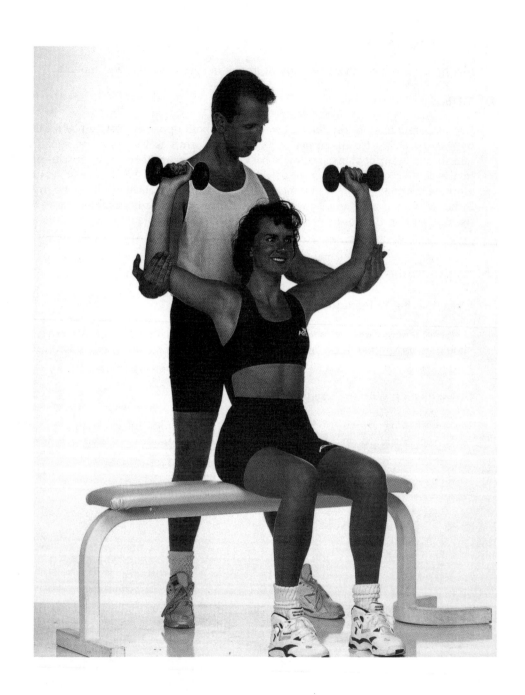

I. Basic Principles, Definitions and Recommendations

All Standards and Guidelines outlined as follows apply to an average adult without known physiological or biological conditions that would in any way restrict his/her exercise activities. These Standards and Guidelines are designed to be used in conjunction with the "Basic Exercise Standards and Guidelines of the Aerobics and Fitness Association of America."

A. Terminology

1. Low-impact Aerobics with Low Weight

    Low-impact aerobics is a form of exercise in which all of the movement patterns are performed with one foot in contact with the floor (see "Standards and Guidelines for Non-weighted Low-impact Aerobics," section I) while utilizing a hand-held or wrist-attached low weight. Ankle weights should never be worn during the aerobic portion of a class.

2. Low Weight

    For the purpose of teaching group exercise, low weight refers to exercising with a weight load of 20 pounds or less. The amount of weight recommended is dependent upon the type of workout and the variables involved with each type. See chart: Training Principles and Guidelines located in this chapter for appropriate weight recommendations.

3. Fixed Resistance

    Exercises are designed to strengthen specific muscles by causing them to overcome a fixed resistance, usually in the form of a dumbbell, barbell or machine. This allows an individual to work with weights at the greatest load that allows completion of the movement. The amount of weight an individual can lift is limited by the strength of the weakest muscle performing the particular exercise. This means that the force generated by the muscles during a contraction is not maximum throughout all phases of the movement.

4. Variable Resistance

Variable resistance is performed on a machine designed to accommodate varying degrees of muscle strength within the full range of motion of an exercise. Variable resistance attempts to coordinate the mechanical advantage of joint position with increased force by using a series of metal cams or other devices to adjust the resistance in accordance with the lever capabilities of a specific joint movement. An individual is capable of performing both concentric and eccentric contractions. The limiting factor of variable resistance machines is that only one muscle group can be isolated at a time.

5. Progressive Resistance Exercise

Progressive resistance exercise is the basis for all weight training programs and is the practical application of the overload principle. As muscle strength improves, it's necessary to periodically increase the amount of resistance so strength improvements will continue.

6. Circuit Training

Circuit training is a method generally utilized to increase cardiovascular fitness while performing strength training exercises. Upper and lower extremities are usually alternated in a sequential manner for a designated time, with heart rates monitored at 55-85% of estimated maximum heart rate. Between 8 and 15 exercise stations are commonly used. Exercises chosen are those that isolate all major muscle groups specific to a goal or sport. A circuit is repeated 2-3 times to equal 20-30 minutes of continuous exercise. A circuit may also include cardiovascular equipment as alternate stations to a strength training station.

7. Interval Training

Interval training refers to high-intensity, intermittent exercise in which repeated exercise bouts of a given intensity are alternated with a relief interval (either rest-relief or work-relief). The intensity and duration of the exercise interval, the length and type of relief interval, and the number of intervals can be modified depending on desired outcome.

B. Who Should Use Low Weights

Low weights are used in exercise programs to provide resistance for muscular strengthening and, when used with low-impact aerobics, cardiovascular conditioning and muscle endurance training. Healthy individuals without a known history of cardiorespiratory conditions, hypertension or joint injury may safely participate in a weighted workout. Sedentary individuals beginning an exercise program should not use weights in a low-impact setting until they can complete a non-weighted workout including a variety of speeds, full range of motion activities and demonstrate the ability to create and work against resistance (see section II.D of this chapter). Persons currently participating in a non-weighted exercise program, who have a history of joint problems or other orthopedic limitations, should consult their physician prior to attempting weighted exercise. For important precautions and contraindications, see "Basic Exercise Standards and Guidelines," section IV.

C. Who Should Not Use Low Weights

Exercise with low weights is not recommended for persons with known cardiovascular disease, with a history of high blood pressure or for those who are at an increased risk of stroke, heart attack or hypertension. The increased peripheral vascular resistance that can occur with weights causes an increase in both systolic and diastolic blood pressure. Weighted workouts are also not recommended for individuals with musculoskeletal limitations, joint injuries, muscle strains, tendinitis, bursitis or ligamentitis, unless specifically ordered by a physician for rehabilitative purposes.

D. When To Use Weights

1. Hand-held or attached wrist weights may be used for upper body strenthening exercises in a stationary position.

2. Hand-held or attached weights may be used in low-impact cardiovascular conditioning workouts.

3. Ankle weights may be used for lower body strengthening in a stationary position.

E. When Not To Use Weights

1. Weights should not be used during pre-aerobic warm-up or post-aerobic cool-down.

2. Neither hand-held weights nor ankle weights should be used while performing high-impact moves.

3. Weights should not be used to perform fast movements which rely on force or momentum.

4. Weights should not be used on a limb that has been injured unless specifically performed for rehabilitative purposes under a physician's supervision.

F. Types of Low Weights

1. Dumbbell or stick-type

2. Wraparound or slip-on weights used on ankles or wrists and secured by Velcro straps; may be held in hand. Some models provide capacity to add weights in small increments.

3. Weighted gloves contain weights in pockets on back and/or in palm of hand.

G. How To Hold/Attach Weights

1. Hand-held weights should be positioned comfortably in palm of hand. Grip weights lightly. When weight is gripped too tightly, blood flow may be restricted (increased peripheral vascular resistance) and tendons in the forearm may be injured.

2. Wraparound weights should be securely fastened so they do not slip and cause friction, but not so tight that blood flow is constricted.

H. How Much Weight

The following ranges provide a minimum and maximum weight that may be safely and effectively used in a low-weight class setting. Heavier weights may be used on an individual basis under the direction of a qualified trainer. Persons beginning to work with weights should use the lower weight recommended for each given range.

1. Upper body work in a stationary position: 1-20 lbs.

2. Low-impact cardiovascular conditioning: 1/2-3 lbs.

3. Lower body leg work: 1/2-10 lbs. depending on muscle group. See individual guidelines for each muscle group in sections IX-XIV of this chapter.

I. When To Increase Weight

An individual should not add weight until she/he can perform 2 sets of 8 repetitions in the same range of motion without fatiguing the muscle(s) (see section II.B-C of this chapter).

When using low weights for cardiovascular conditioning, the added resistance may increase heart rate. Heart rate should be within an individual's training heart rate range for the duration of the activity.

Training Principles and Guidelines				
Type of Activity	Frequency	Duration	Intensity	Amount of Wt.
Type I Class Weights are used for low-impact cardiovascular conditioning and both upper and lower body strengthening.	3-4 x per week	60-90 min., including 25-35 min. for low- impact portion	55-85% of estimated maximum HR	1/2-3 lbs. for low-impact; 1-20 lbs. for upper and lower body, depending on muscle group and type of weight
Type II Class Weights are used only for upper and lower body strengthening. Aerobic training is accomplished elsewhere.	2-4 x per week, depending upon amount of weight	Minimum of 20 min. for upper body; minimum of 20 min. for lower body	55-90% of estimated maximum HR	1-20 lbs. for upper and lower body, depending on muscle group and type of weight
Type III Class Weights are used for upper and lower body strengthening, but not during cardiovascular portion of class.	3-5 x per week, depending upon amount of weight	60-90 min., including 20-45 min. for cardiovascular section and 10-30 min. for strengthening	55-85% of estimated maximum HR	No wts. for aerobics; 1-20 lbs. for upper and lower body, depending on muscle group and type of weight
Type IV Class Weights are used in conjunction with non-weighted aerobics or anaerobic intervals as either a timed interval, timed circuit or for active rest.	2-4 x per week	Timed either for intervals or circuits, 30 sec. to 5 min.	55-90% of estimated maximum HR	No wts. for aerobics; 1-10 lbs. for strengthening

II. Training Principles and Guidelines

A. Frequency

1. Weighted workouts are performed in a variety of combinations and formats. The frequency of the workout is based on the type of class. All workouts should be of sufficient frequency to maintain or improve fitness levels, yet avoid potential risk of overuse.

2. Individuals utilizing low weight in conjunction with low-impact aerobics, who want to increase their frequency of workouts to more than 3-4 days per week, should supplement a weighted program with other forms of aerobic exercise without weights.

3. The number of days spent specifically training for strength is dependent upon the amount of weight used. Training with 1-20 pound weights for either upper or lower body can be performed 2-4 days per week. When training with 10-20 pound weights, maintain non-consecutive workout days for upper and lower body as well as alternate muscle groups worked. For example, train upper body 2 days per week and lower body 2 days per week.

4. In addition to alternating body parts, for optimal strength training, also vary weight used to create heavy and light workout days.

B. Intensity

The intensity of a weighted workout for both the aerobic and strengthening portions are controlled by, but not limited to, the following factors: speed of movement, elevated movements, exercise selection, exercise sequencing and movement patterns, lever length, amount of resistance and number of reps and sets per exercise. These factors are interrelated and have a direct effect on each other.

1. Speed

   a. Speed of movement when using weights influences the intensity of the movement and will cause heart rate elevation.

   b. Speed of movement should be appropriate for type of activity being performed, e.g., low-impact aerobics with low weight as opposed to stationary strengthening. Speed should be adapted to amount of weight being used.

   c. The speed of any movement should be performed through a full range of motion in a controlled manner with resistance (see "Basic Exercise Standards and Guidelines," section I.F-G).

   d. Speed of movement during low-impact aerobics, either in place or in traveling patterns across the floor, is appropriate if momentum and alignment are controlled.

   e. Maximum music speed recommended for weighted low-impact aerobics is 140 bpm, with a recommended range of 116-136.

   f. Maximum music speed recommended for weighted muscle strengthening is 134 bpm, with a recommended range of 110-130.

2. Elevated Movements

a. The intensity of a particular movement is influenced by the elevation at which it is performed. Movements that are performed through a full range of motion, requiring extension in either an elevated position and/or out and away from the body, are more intense when using low weights and are thus more difficult to execute and control while maintaining proper body alignment. Such movements should not be considered beginning exercises.

b. Elevated, full range of motion exercises should be comfortably performed, maintaining correct body alignment before additional weight resistance is attempted.

c. To prevent overuse injury, intersperse elevated movements with lower, short lever movements using the same muscle groups.

3. Exercise Selection

a. The variety of movements used and choice of exercise appropriate for an individual's fitness level will be determining factors in raising or lowering exercise intensity as well as maintaining a consistent intensity level throughout the aerobic portion of the class.

b. Exercises should be appropriate for the amount of weight being utilized in the activity, whether choreography calls for movement or a stationary position.

c. Exercises should be selected according to the goals of the program.

4. Movement Sequencing and Patterns

a. In a weighted low-impact class, the intensity can be increased by varying the elevations of arm and leg combinations.

b. Traveling across the floor as part of a continuous pattern will further increase the intensity of a workout, particularly while moving and using a low weight. The amount of traveling and type of movement sequencing are dependent upon class goals and amount of weight being utilized.

5. Lever Length

a. Working with extended levers, e.g., arms and legs, will increase the workload to a particular joint, especially when weight is added.

b. To prevent injury, long lever movements should be interspersed with shorter lever movements or modified, depending upon amount of weight being used. There is a direct relationship between lever length and applied joint stress.

6. Amount of Resistance

a. The amount of resistance being used is dependent upon fitness levels of students, type of program, as well as goals of the program.

b. As the amount of resistance increases, intensity of the program will increase.

c. Avoid using speed with long lever and/or full range of motion movements as the amount of resistance increases.

7. Number of Reps and Sets

    a. The number of reps and sets is dependent upon fitness levels, weight load, exercise selection and program goals. For goals of muscular endurance and definition, use 15-30 repetitions.

    b. As the amount of overload or resistance increases, decrease reps and sets, building up again slowly.

C. Duration

1. A cardiovascular conditioning session utilizing 1/2 to 3-pound weights should meet the minimum criteria of 20-45 minutes in length, not including warm-up or post-aerobic cool-down, set as a standard for achieving a training effect (see "Basic Exercise Standards and Guidelines," sections I.B and VI.B. Also see "Standards and Guidelines for Non-weighted Low-impact Aerobics," section II.C).

2. Muscle strengthening should include sufficient time to overload muscle/muscle groups to produce a training effect. Amount of time spent on each activity is dependent upon the amount of weight, exercise selection and number of repetitions per exercise.

D. Overload

A training effect will occur when a muscle is regularly overloaded beyond the level to which it is accustomed to working (see "Basic Exercise Standards and Guidelines," section I.B). Overload is accomplished by increasing any one or a combination of the following factors: amount of weight, reps, sets and/or intensity with any of the variables listed above in section II.B of this chapter.

1. During a weighted, low-impact aerobics class, when using appropriate weight, resistance, speed and range of motion, a *minimum* of 2 sets of 8 repetitions per set of the same movement should be sufficient to fatigue the muscle or muscle group being worked.

2. For a strengthening non-aerobic workout, overload is best achieved by progressively increasing the amount of weight, or the number of reps and sets per muscle group as the workload becomes easier. The training method of overload used is dependent upon training goals, e.g., muscle strength vs. muscle endurance (hypertrophy vs. tone).

3. Performing a high number of repetitions with low weight will increase muscle endurance and definition. Performing a small number of repetitions with heavier weight will hypertrophy muscle fibers and increase strength. Using high repetition with low weights while moving in a weighted low-impact class will additionally increase cardiovascular conditioning.

E. Resistance

Whether one is working with or without the added resistance of weights, muscle strengthening occurs when a muscle or group of muscles is worked against a resistance (see "Basic Exercise Standards and Guidelines," section I.F). To achieve maximum effectiveness, resistance is accomplished not only by the use of weights, but by controlling the amount of tension during both the concentric and eccentric phase of a movement.

Recruitment of muscle fiber is increased as a muscle and/or muscle group becomes "trained," increasing the amount of tension or force that the muscle(s) must work against. This type of "consciously applied resistance" is only possible if movements are performed in a controlled manner at a slow to moderate pace.

F. Isolation and Specificity

When training with weights, it is important to:

1. Identify your goals and the focus of each of your exercises, e.g., strengthening thighs for a skier; toning the neglected upper body of a runner; or providing a comprehensive strengthening regimen.

2. Identify the muscle or muscle groups being strengthened.

3. Choose exercises that will specifically isolate and work the muscles that are the focus of your workout goals.

4. Remember to work the opposing muscle(s) to avoid muscular imbalance (see "Basic Exercise Standards and Guidelines," section I.D).

G. Exercise Danger Signs When Using Low Weights and Other General Precautions

1. Know the Exercise Danger Signs outlined in "Basic Exercise Standards and Guidelines," section III.A. In addition, be aware of the following conditions and considerations and understand their relationship to the added physiological stresses of working with weights.

    a. Momentum—never let a weight build up momentum because the risk of joint and muscle injury is increased.

    b. Breathing and the Valsalva maneuver—see "Basic Exercise Standards and Guidelines," section IV.E.

    c. Effect of lever length on joint stress—the longer the lever the greater the resistance, increasing risk of injury in and around the joint.

    d. Hyperextension of the joints—tendency to hyperextend increases with weighted exercise; limb and joint injury occurs with hyperextension along with weakening of ligaments, tendons and connective tissue.

    e. Too much weight/inappropriate weight for activity—overstresses muscles and joints.

    f. High-impact movement—not recommended for weighted workouts.

    g. Heart rate—see "Basic Exercise Standards and Guidelines," sectionVI.I, for when and how to determine heart rate.

H. Posture and Alignment

See "Basic Exercise Standards and Guidelines," section I.D-E. In addition, be aware of the danger of locking or hyperextending joints, and the added joint and ligament stress of weighted workouts.

I. Breathing

Breathing rhythmically throughout exercise is essential to preventing blood pressure and heart rate elevation. Exhaling on the exertion will help prevent over-elevation (see "Basic Exercise Standards and Guidelines," section IV.E).

Ill. Class Format

A. Select Type of Class According to Training Principles and Guidelines Chart Following Section I in This Chapter.

B. Considerations Specific to a Weighted Aerobic Workout

1. Performing specific stationary resistive arm or leg work immediately prior to performing aerobics may make arm or leg movements during aerobics difficult to perform due to muscle fatigue and lactic acid build-up.

2. Working a muscle or muscle group to maximum effort for significant strength gains is not possible with a light weight, particularly while moving.

3. The intensity of a weighted cardiovascular workout is dependent upon: a) an individual's ability to use resistance while moving and b) the variables listed in section II.B of this chapter.

C. Sequence

The following is the recommended sequence as adapted by AFAA for a one-hour weighted class:

1. Pre-class instruction

2. Warm-up with no weights. Warm-up should be specific to weighted activities being performed.

3. Cardiovascular conditioning and post-aerobic cooldown if Class Type I, II or IV (see Training Principles and Guidelines Chart following section I in this chapter)

4. Standing muscular strengthening work for upper and/or lower body in any of the recommended positions for each category

5. Floorwork for muscular strengthening, in order of preference:

    a. Legs

    b. Buttocks

    c. Abdominals

    d. Lower back

6. Static stretching

IV. Pre-Class Procedure

A. Instructor Checklist

Review points to cover in "Basic Exercise Standards and Guidelines," section IV:

1. Medical clearance
2. Level of participation
3. Appropriate shoes
4. Breathing
5. Aerobics orientation

B. Orientation to the Use of Low Weights

Review the following information with students as necessary:

1. Why use weights
2. Who **should** use weights
3. Who should **not** use weights
4. When the class will use weights
5. Types of weights class will use and proper method of use and attachment
6. How much weight to use
7. When it is necessary to increase weight
8. How to create resistance
9. Importance of body alignment and how to avoid joint and ligament injury

V. Warm-Up

A. Purpose

Prepares the body for vigorous exercise and may reduce the risk of injury.

B. Time

A 10 to 15-minute warm-up period is recommended.

C. Method for a Weighted Workout

1. Warm-up should consist of a balanced combination of static stretches and smoothly performed, rhythmic limbering exercises, in addition to joint preparatory exercises that will further ready the upper torso joints and muscles for the increased stress of a weighted workout.

2. The guidelines for warm-up sequencing, muscle groups utilized, rhythmic limbering exercise and static stretching, and special do's and don'ts, described in "Basic Exercise Standards and Guidelines," section V, should be followed.

VI. Cardiovascular Conditioning with Low Weights

A. Training Effect

Significant improvements of the biochemical and cellular levels of the aerobic transport system have been shown to occur with high repetition/low-weight work. In addition, if heart rate is maintained in the 55-85% training heart rate range, cardiovascular conditioning, as achieved in other forms of aerobic exercise, will also occur.

B. Time

20-45 minutes is recommended.

C. Sequence Using Low Weights

1. Start slowly and gradually increase the intensity and range of motion of your movements. All considerations discussed in "Basic Exercise Standards and Guidelines," section VI.C, should be observed until a steady state has been achieved (approximately 3-5 minutes after the aerobic portion has begun).

2. Low-impact aerobics should be maintained when exercising with low weights (see "Standards and Guidelines for Non-weighted Low-impact Aerobics," section VI.B).

3. Heart rate should be maintained at 55-85% of estimated maximum heart rate (see "Basic Exercise Standards and Guidelines," section VI.I, for calculation and monitoring methods). Heart rate is elevated or decreased by regulating the intensity of the exercise. Factors include:

   a. Elevation of movement

   b. Specific, resistive movements

   c. Amount of weight

   d. Speed

   e. Range of motion

   f. Movement sequencing and patterning

D. Precautions When Using Weights

1. 1/2-3 pound hand-held or attached wrist weights may be used during low-impact aerobics.

2. AFAA strongly recommends ankle weights not be worn during the aerobic conditioning segment. The specific stress of added weight on ankles may create the potential for overuse injuries such as stress fractures, tendinitis, compartment syndrome or shin splints. The injury potential increases as the impact pressure

increases per square inch. Additionally, posture alignment could be altered, resulting in stress to the lumbar spine and the knees.

3. Increased muscular compression during contraction can occlude blood flow within the vessels. Compromised circulation adds additional risk to those with high blood pressure or those at risk of cardiovascular injury or stroke.

4. Skin chafing and irritation can occur when weights are not securely fastened. It is recommended to place ankle weights over socks when using them for stationary lower body strengthening.

5. It is a common mistake to hold one's breath while working with weights. Holding one's breath while "bearing down" causes the Valsalva maneuver, increasing the possibility for fainting, lightheadedness or irregular heart rhythm.

VII. Post-Aerobic Cool-down

A. Purpose

The post-aerobic cool-down provides a transition period between vigorous aerobic work and less taxing exercise, allowing working heart rate to return safely to pre-exercise rate without overstressing the cardiovascular system.

B. Time

3-5 minutes is recommended.

C. Type of Movement

Rhythmic movement that gradually decreases in speed and range of motion should be utilized with or without weights, depending upon exercise selection.

D. Method

1. See "Standards and Guidelines for Non-weighted Low-impact Aerobics," section VII.D, if weights are not utilized as part of cool-down progression.

2. Specific weighted work for either upper or lower body can be utilized as part of the post-aerobic cool-down as long as cardiovascular conditioning has ceased and heart rate reduction guidelines are being met.

3. If weights are used as part of the post-aerobic cool-down, complete the progression with rhythmic limbering and static stretching without weights for major muscle groups (see "Standards and Guidelines for Non-weighted Low-impact Aerobics," section VII.D).

VIII. Upper Body Exercises

A. Purpose

To strengthen the muscles of the upper body: arms, chest, shoulders and back.

B. Time

8-30 minutes is recommended, depending upon class type.

C. Alignment

1. Maintain neutral pelvic alignment for all positions utilized.
2. Keep shoulders relaxed.
3. Don't lean forward or backward in a standing position.
4. Joints should not hyperextend (lock); keep knees slightly flexed.
5. Use good posture as recommended in "Basic Exercise Standards and Guidelines," section I.E.

D. Method

1. Work opposing muscle groups for muscle balance.
2. Specific sequence is not critical when working with 3 pounds or less, but strive for a complete upper body workout.
3. When using heavier weights, strengthen larger muscle groups first.
4. Movements should be smooth, controlled, resistive and slow enough to allow for complete extension. Momentum should not be used as work is not effectively accomplished and a potential for joint injury is created.
5. Alternate arm work performed above shoulder height with arm work done below shoulder height. This will maximize effectiveness of specific muscle group work and decrease muscle fatigue caused by holding weighted arms above shoulders for too long.
6. Use a variety of positions that will optimize muscle work against gravity.

IX. Lower Body Muscle Strengthening

A. Purpose

To strengthen the muscles of the abdomen and lower body.

B. Time

10-20 minutes is recommended, depending upon type of class.

C. Sequence

1. In a one-hour class that includes cardiorespiratory conditioning, it is often difficult to include all muscle groups during this section, particularly if the aerobic segment exceeds 20 minutes. If time is a problem, alternate muscle groups with each session, e.g., one day do quadriceps, buttocks and hamstrings, the next session do inner and outer thighs and calves. Include abdominal exercises at each session.

2. Lower body exercises may be performed in order of preference.

3. Lower body strengthening may be performed in a variety of positions, e.g., side-lying, prone, supine or standing.

4. Other equipment or attachments, such as rubber bands, elastic tubing or weighted balls, may be substituted for an attached or hand-held weight as long as the joints and muscles involved are safely moved through a full range of motion while utilizing the alternative equipment.

5. If alternative equipment is selected, it should be appropriate to the activity and fitness level of the students.

D. General Recommendations

1. Use appropriate weight recommended for each muscle group.

2. Heart rate should always be at 60% or less of estimated maximum heart rate when performing floorwork.

3. Avoid using momentum, or jerking or throwing movements; movements should be controlled and resistive.

4. Do not hyperextend joints or lower back.

5. Isolate the muscle(s) that are the primary focus of the exercise.

6. See sections X-XIV of this chapter for specific recommendations for isolated muscle groups.

X. Abdominals

A. Purpose

To strengthen the abdominal muscles: rectus abdominis and the external and internal oblique muscles.

B. Time

4-8 minutes is recommended.

C. Method

1. General considerations should follow those outlined in "Basic Exercise Standards and Guidelines," section XI.

2. The amount of weight used, either hand-held or attached to ankles, should not exceed 3 pounds.

3. When using hand-held weights, position them either on the chest or close to the body. Never do abdominal work while holding weights above or behind head.

4. Weights may be attached to the ankles for the purpose of abdominal strengthening when leg movement is also included. See "Basic Exercise Standards and Guidelines," section XI.E, regarding abdominal vs. hip flexor exercises.

5. Avoid throwing the upper body forward or relying on momentum.

6. Support the head if needed.

7. Exercises for both the rectus abdominis and oblique muscles should be included.

8. Standing abdominal work or "waist work" is not the most effective means for strengthening the oblique muscles. If standing waist work is performed, it should be in a slow, controlled manner with the lower body in a stationary position to protect the erector spinae and other muscles that attach to the spine and pelvic girdle.

XI. Hip Abductor and Hip Adductor

A. Purpose

To strengthen the muscles of the outer and inner thigh (gluteus medius), adductor group, pectineus and gracilis.

B. Time

10-15 minutes is recommended.

C. Method

1. Alignment, method and injury prevention recommendations follow those described in "Basic Exercise Standards and Guidelines," section IX. C-F.

2. The recommended weight for attached ankle weights is 3 pounds.

3. Supine adductor work should be performed with the knees slightly bent and not more than shoulder width apart. Movement should resist toward the midline of body. If this position is used with ankle weights attached, the lower back must remain on the floor throughout the exercise. Legs should be extended in the air as close to being perpendicular to the hips as possible.

4. In order to avoid allowing stronger quadriceps to perform work of hip abductors or adductors, do not roll backward when in the side-lying position.

5. The long-lying position with head relaxed on forearm is the recommended position if ankle weight is attached.

6. Abducting in the all-fours position is not recommended due to the difficulty it poses with added weight. Additionally, the "L" position, in which the legs are at a 90-degree angle to the torso, may cause excessive strain to the gluteus medius tendon and

should be avoided. Hip circles should also be avoided because of the potential for joint injury.

7. Hip abduction and adduction exercises can also be performed in a standing position as long as good posture and alignment are utilized. Weights may be placed on the ankles as long as there is no impact involved. However, if a side leg lift is combined, for example, with a squat, weights should not be attached to ankles due to impact of movement. Instead, weights may be hand-held, supported on shoulders or waist.

8. Hand-held weights should not exceed 10 pounds.

XII. Quadriceps Group

A. Purpose

To strengthen the quadriceps muscles: rectus femoris and vastus group.

B. Time

5-8 minutes is recommended.

C. Method

1. Basic alignment and considerations are the same as those outlined in "Basic Exercise Standards and Guidelines," section IX.J-K.

2. There are a number of positions that may be utilized: supine, sitting or standing. The position used for exercises that involve hip flexion and/or knee extension will be dependent upon the student's strength and ability to maintain the position with proper alignment while performing the exercise.

3. Amount of weight recommended is 1-20 pounds if hand-held and 1-10 pounds if attached, depending upon position, fitness level and exercise selection.

4. Number of reps and sets will be dependent upon the variables listed above in section XII.C,2 of this chapter, as well as amount of weight.

5. Medially or laterally rotating the hips will determine which muscle(s) of the quadriceps group is(are) being isolated and emphasized.

6. Hand-held weights, placed either on shoulders or waist, may be used for standing squats and lunges. Upper body strengthening may be incorporated as long as proper body alignment can be maintained throughout exercise. Avoid using ankle weights when performing squats and lunges or any other similar variations when the lower body is bearing weight.

7. When performing a squat and any variation of the squat, feet may be placed shoulder width apart, or slightly more than shoulder width apart, with knees relaxed. Squat in a controlled manner, lowering torso until thighs are parallel or slightly above parallel to the floor. At no time should hips drop below knee level, causing hyperflexion of the knee. From the squat position, straighten legs using strong

quadriceps extension. Keep lower back flat and fixed during the entire descent and ascent to reduce overstraining of back muscles.

8. When performing a lunge and any variation of the lunge, the front knee should never "overshoot" toes. This places tremendous strain on the knee joint and its attachments. Therefore, the lower front leg should be perpendicular to the heel during any lunge position. Depth of the lunge will vary, depending on type of lunge being performed. However, a lunge should never be so low that knee pain or strain is felt.

9. When performing standing or supine knee extensions, do not hyperextend or lock knee. The exercise should be performed in a controlled manner without any rapid, jerky movements.

XIII. Hamstring Group and Buttocks

A. Purpose

To strengthen the buttocks and rear thigh muscles: gluteus maximus and hamstring group.

B. Time

5-8 minutes is recommended.

C. Method

1. Basic alignment and considerations are the same as those outlined in "Basic Exercise Standards and Guidelines," section IX-L.

2. Amount of weight recommended is 1-20 pounds if hand-held, 1-10 pounds if attached.

3. Hamstring strengthening is best accomplished by assuming a position on all fours (hands and knees or elbows and knees) or lying prone on the stomach. Heel is pulled with controlled resistance toward buttocks.

4. When using ankle weights and performing exercises for the gluteus maximus, the movements are easier to control if performed on elbows and knees as opposed to hands and knees. Arching the lower back, thrusting the leg, and performing movements that rely on momentum should be avoided.

5. Longer lever movements should be avoided (or poundage reduced) if alignment cannot be maintained when using a weight.

6. Buttocks and hamstring strengthening may also be performed in a standing position. Using a wall or other support is recommended when performing knee flexion and hip extension exercises in a standing position to help maintain proper body alignment. Ankle weights may be attached if no impact is involved.

7. Squats and lunges may be performed for hamstring and buttocks strengthening if emphasis is on the upward or ascending portion of the movement (see guidelines and position recommendations in previous section XII.C,7-8 of this chapter).

XIV. Lower Leg Strengthening

A. Purpose

To strengthen the calf muscles and muscles on the front of the shin: gastrocnemius, soleus and tibialis anterior.

B. Time

5-8 minutes is recommended.

C. Method

1. Exercises for strengthening calf muscles usually involve controlled heel raises, using one or both legs at a time, with or without a weight. Knees are bent or straight, depending upon which calf muscle is being isolated.

2. Amount of weight recommended is 1-20 pounds if hand-held.

3. A wall or other support may be necessary for balance with some exercise variations, particularly when holding a weight.

4. Maintain good posture and alignment as recommended for standing postural alignment in "Basic Exercise Standards and Guidelines," section I.E.

5. To work the calves effectively, press completely up onto the ball of the foot. Body weight must be balanced over the ball of the foot and maintained throughout the lifting and lowering phases of the exercise.

6. Balance muscle groups to prevent injury by including exercises for both calf and shin muscles.

7. To work the front of the lower leg, weights may be placed on ankles or across the top of the foot, in a non-impact situation. In this position and using control, dorsi-flex foot toward head.

XV. Cool-Down Stretches

A. Purpose

To increase flexibility and relieve any metabolic waste accumulated in muscles from strengthening exercises.

B. Time

4-7minutes at the end of class is recommended.

C. Method

1. All considerations outlined in "Basic Exercise Standards and Guidelines," section XII.A-G, should be adhered to.

2. Weights should not be utilized during the cool-down period.

References

Abrams, D.E. (July/August, 1984). AFAA reports on aerobic injury research. *American Fitness*, 2.

Aerobics & Fitness Association of America (April, 1988). Walking with weights. *American Fitness*, 6.

Angston, P. (September, 1987). Low-impact aerobics comes of age. *American Fitness*, 5.

Astrand, P.-O., & Rodahl, K. (1970). Textbook work physiology. New York: McGraw-Hill Co.

Bartell, P. (May/June, 1986). Take time: A new pace for exercise. *American Fitness*, 4.

Benmore, L. (October, 1988). Achieving continuity in your aerobic workout. *American Fitness*, 6.

Brewster, C. (September/October, 1984). Make a great comeback: Latest advice on making a post-injury recovery. *American Fitness*, 2.

Carroll, J. (May/June, 1988). Injuries in low-impact and high-impact aerobic dance. *American Fitness*, 6.

Carroll, J. (January/February, 1986). Misalignment. *American Fitness*, 4.

Cautwell, J.D. (October, 1984). The legacy of jim fixx. *American Fitness*, 2.

Choi, J. (September/October, 1984). Sudden death in jogging under the age of forty. *American Fitness*, 2.

Clippinger-Robertson, K. (November/December, 1985). Prevention of low back injuries. *American Fitness*, 3.

Cohen, L., & Sukov, R. (September/October, 1984). Stress fractures: How do we know? *American Fitness*, 2.

Cooper, P. (Ed.) (1985). Aerobics: Theory and practice. Sherman Oaks: Aerobics and Fitness Association of America.

Falsetti, H.L., & Proudfit, S.O. (September/October, 1985). Injury rate report for aerobic instructors. *American Fitness*, 3.

Ferrari, M.B. (January/February, 1987). Spice up your classes with variety training: Circuit aerobics. *American Fitness*, 5.

Hatfield, F. (1983). Aerobic weight training. Chicago: Contemporary Books.

Johnson, S. (April, 1988). Deep in the heart of fitness. *American Fitness*, 6.

McArdle, W.D., Katch, F.I., & Katch, V.L. (1986). Exercise physiology. Philadelphia: Lea & Febiger.

Pink, M., & Terrell, S. (July/August, 1984). Aerobic injury questionnaire. *American Fitness*, 2.

Price, J. (October, 1987). Interview with james garrick, a peak condition advisor. *American Fitness*, 5.

Rasch, P.J., & Burke, R.K. (1963). Kinesiology and applied anatomy. Philadelphia: Lea & Febiger.

Rosenberg, S.L. (October, 1987). Aerobic dance injuries: Why me? *American Fitness*, 5.

Schnack, M. (March/April, 1986). Sports injuries: No longer an end to exercising. *American Fitness*, 4.

Scott, N., Nisonsson, B., & Nicholas, J. (Eds.) (1984). Principles of sports medicine. Baltimore/London: Williams & Wilkins.

Sukov, R.J., & Cohen, L.J. (November/December, 1984). Diagnostic ultrasound: Seeing with soundwaves. *American Fitness*, 2.

Voeller, S. (January/February, 1988). One, two, buckle your shoe. *American Fitness*, 6.

Watterson, C. (October, 1987). Does instructor training reduce injury rates? *American Fitness*, 5.

Wolkodoff, N. (July/August, 1989). Building strength. *IDEA Today*, 7:7.

Yeager, T. (November/December, 1984). Get more from your workout. *American Fitness*, 2.

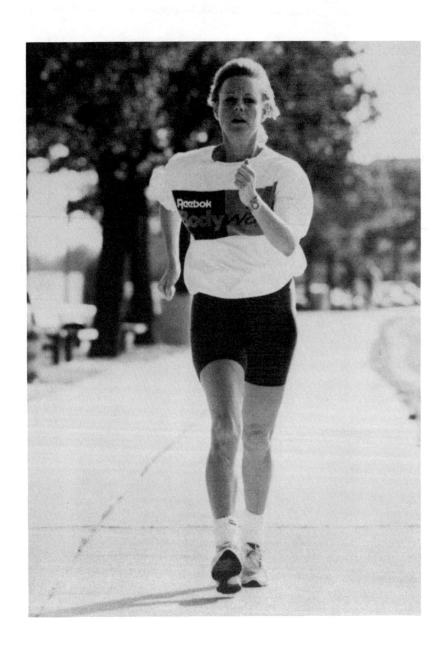

Walk Reebok Technique

I. Body Alignment and Walk Reebok^{SM} Training

Good body alignment is important in the prevention of sport and exercise related injuries. Instructors should continually remind participants to maintain appropriate posture when performing all bodywalk techniques.

The primary focus when performing Walk Reebok Technique I is on posture. Therefore, the following techniques should be emphasized:

1. Head in the neutral position (head centered, chin parallel to the ground, eyes looking ahead).

2. Shoulders down, pulled back and relaxed.

3. Chest lifted.

4. Abdominals contracted and buttocks tucked under the hips.

5. Arms relaxed and swinging in opposition to the legs.

6. Maintain a comfortable stride.

When performing Walk Reebok Technique II the primary focus is on the arm swing and foot roll. Therefore, the following techniques should be emphasized:

1. Maintain good posture.

2. Flex the elbows to approximately 90 degrees. The forward swing should not cross the center of the body or swing higher than the top of the sternum.

3. Speed up the arm swing to speed up the leg action.

4. The hips rotate slightly (this is a natural motion).

5. Land on the heel of the foot with the forefoot raised.

6. Forcefully push off the forefoot.

7. Lean slightly forward from the ankles, not the hips.

When performing Walk Reebok Technique III steps will become slightly longer but much quicker, the hips will rotate forward and backward and the placement of the foot will form a continuous straight line with the inner edges of the feet. Therefore, the following techniques should be emphasized:

1. Maintain good posture.

2. Drive the elbows back on the arm swing (hand should not reach farther back than the buttocks).

3. Increase the speed of the arm swing.

4. Rotate the hips forward and backward.

5. Place the feet closer to a straight line (almost like tightrope walking).

6. Forcefully push the forefoot against the ground.

7. Keep the ball of the rear foot on the ground until the heel of the forward leg has contacted the ground.

8. Lean forward from the ankles, not the hips.

II. Segments of a Walk Reebok Class

Each Walk Reebok class should be divided into 4 segments-a warm-up and stretch, aerobic walking, isolation work and post or slow stretch.

A. Warm-Up

The purpose of the warm-up is to prepare the body for exercise by:

1. Increasing the internal body temperature by 1 or 2 degrees.

2. Increasing blood flow to the muscles.

3. Reducing the risk of cardiac complications (electrocardiographic abnormalities).

The **warm-up** should consist of a rhythmic, full range of motion activities such as leisurely walking (Walk Reebok Technique I) approximately 5 minutes in duration. After the body has been warmed, the **stretch** portion should include 6 to 8 minutes of static stretching exercises (working from head to toe), each held for at least 10 seconds.

B. Stretch

The purpose of the stretch is to:

1. Increase joint range of motion.

2. Increase muscle elasticity

3. Reduce the risk of musculoskeletal injury.

III. Aerobic walking

The purpose of the aerobic walking is to improve specific aspects of health such as:

1. Improves aerobic fitness.
2. Reduces risk for cardiovascular disease.
3. Reduces percent of body fat.
4. Increases bone density.
5. Improves psychological well-being.

Specific to each technique:

1. Walk Reebok I, a leisurely form of walking, can reduce the risk of heart disease and osteoporosis, enhance feelings of well-being and improve body composition.
2. Walk Reebok II is designed to increase aerobic fitness and caloric expenditure.
3. Walk Reebok III, a more advanced technique, provides participants with a greater challenge and increased caloric expenditure.

IV. Isolation work

The purpose of isolation work is to strengthen key areas of the body not adequately exercised during the aerobic segment. The rationale for strengthening specific muscles is to:

1. Help muscles resist potentially injurious mechanical stresses.
2. Restore and maintain muscle balance to promote proper posture and good body mechanics.
3. Enhance Walk Reebok performance.
4. Improve body composition and thus physical appearance.

Isolation work should consist of safe and effective strength exercises, using 2 to 3 sets of 8 to 16 repetitions with appropriate resistance.

V. Slow stretch

The purpose of the slow stretch is to elongate the muscles that have been contracting through a limited range of motion during the walking segment and to improve overall flexibility, facilitating the performance of daily activities. The slow stretch should include a variety of stretching exercises, each of which should be held for 10 to 30 seconds.

*Walk Reebok exercise techniques have been reprinted with permission from Reebok International, Ltd.

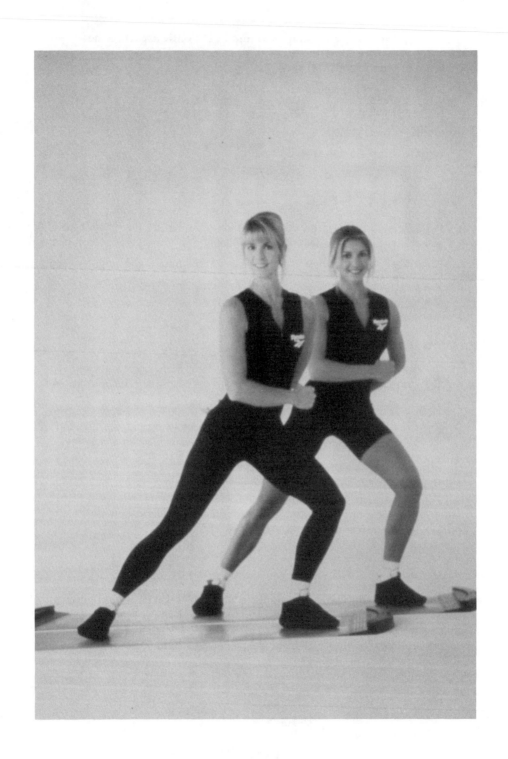

Slide Reebok
Terminology and Guidelines

The information in this section forms the building blocks of Slide Reebok[SM], and establishes the basic vocabulary and principles of the Basic Training program, as well as for the other upcoming programs. The terms will remain consistent from the beginning to the most advanced workouts. Since this information is so critical, we urge you to take as much time as you need to become familiar with it.

I. Terminology

- **Lateral Movement Training**

  Slide training, which utilizes side-to-side motion to specifically train the musculature of the lower body. Over the long term, it may help to protect and strengthen the muscles crossing the joint of the hip, knee and ankle while simultaneously promoting overall fitness.

- **End Ramp**

  The biomechanically positioned and designed end pieces which are used for initiating, ending or stabilizing each movement.

- **Slide Reebok[TM] Sock**

  The covering that slips over an athletic shoe. It reduces friction and facilitates the sliding motion.

A. Body Positions

- **The Front Position**

  In this position, stand facing forward. Start at the end ramp. Keep your feet together, with the foot of your trail leg in contact with the end ramp.

- **The End Position**

  In the end position, you stand sideways, facing the end ramp. Your feet are together, and your toes are on the end ramp.

- **The Center Position**

  In the center position, stand in the center of the board, with your feet together, facing forward.

B. Stances

- ### The Upright Stance

  As its name implies, you remain upright throughout the movement in this stance. Even though your torso is erect, keep a slight bend in your knees. To help your balance, put your hands on your hips, on the top of your thighs or behind your back. Throughout the sliding motion, keep your shoulders over your hips and level with the floor. To maintain balance, keep your weight distributed evenly on both feet.

- ### The Athletic Ready Stance

  This stance has a more pronounced bend in the knee and hip. Until you get used to the sliding motion, loosely relax your hands on the top of your thighs. It will help support your back and maintain your balance. Avoid rolling your shoulders forward or bending from the waist.

C. Leg Positions

- ### Trail Leg

  The leg that is against the end ramp before the move begins. This leg pushes during the initiation of the sliding motion and trails during the glide.

- ### Lead Leg

  The leg farther away from the end ramp. It leads and stabilizes the body during the glide.

D. Workouts

- ### The Athletic Training Track

  These workouts take a sports-oriented approach, and offer an athletic style of training that can be performed without music.

- ### The Rhythmic Training Track

  These workouts utilize music and pay special attention to choreography and combinations that can be performed in a more stylized approach typical of aerobic dance.

II. Guidelines

Every time you or one of your clients trains with Slide Reebok^{SM}, follow these 10 guidelines for proper posture and technique:

1. Approach the board from the back, so that the end ramps angle outward and you can read the logo. For most of the moves, you will begin in the front position, with the foot of your trail leg against one of the end ramps.

2. Center your weight over your feet.

3. Keep the knees aligned with the toes at all times. At no time should the knees extend past the toes.

4. Keep the hips squared and aligned with the torso and shoulders.

5. Keeping a slight bend in the knee, push down and toward the side from the ramp with the muscles on the outside of the hip and leg. Make sure the press comes from the entire thigh and leg, not the foot or ankle, of the trail leg (which is adjacent to the ramp).

6. After you start the slide, control your speed by dragging the trail leg. Use the lead leg only as a stabilizing influence while moving across the board.

7. For the basic slide, bring the trail leg to a closed position before beginning the slide back.

8. Until you are comfortable with the slide, keep your eyes on the board. Gradually get into the habit of keeping the head in neutral alignment with your eyes forward, or look in the direction of the sliding motion.

9. Proceed to the more complex core movements or add arm motions only when you are proficient with the basic slide move.

10. When doing variations, lifts or touches, stabilize and balance yourself on the ramp before initiating the additional movement.

*Guidelines two and four are applicable to the basic slide or while developing proficiency with the core moves.

III. The Warm-Up and Cool-Down

As with any physical activity, reduce your risk of injury by warming up before and cooling down after a workout. Warm up by raising your body temperature with 8 to 12 minutes of light activity. Then stretch the muscles of the lower extremities, including the quadriceps, hamstrings, abductors, adductors, gluteals, gastrocnemius, soleus, peroneals, tibialis anterior and erector spinae. Hold each stretch to mild tension for eight to 12 seconds, without bouncing. In the cool-down section, hold each stretch for a longer period of time.

IV. The Benefits of Slide Reebok Training:

1. Prepares the body for demanding planting and lateral moves with minimal stress.

2. Improves agility and balance.

3. Improves muscle strength.

4. Improves aerobic fitness.

5. Improves percent of body fat through increased caloric expenditure.

*Slide Reebok exercise techniques have been reprinted
with permission from Reebok International, Ltd.

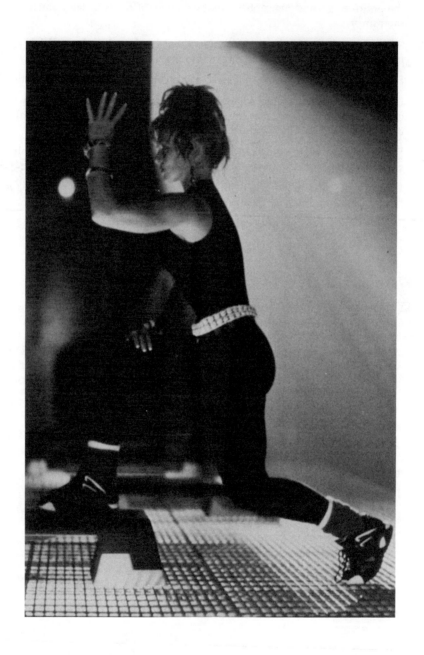

Step Training Technique

To minimize the risk of injury and maximize the conditioning benefits of stepping, teach the following body alignment and stepping technique guidelines to your class participants. Watch them continually to monitor their form, and coach as necessary.

I. Body Alignment

1. Shoulders back and relaxed.
2. Chest lifted and body erect.
3. Abdominals contracted to support torso.
4. Neutral spine.
5. Knees relaxed, not locked.
6. Avoid hyperextension of joints.
7. Avoid twisting or torquing of joints.

II. Stepping Technique

1. Use a full body lean. Do not bend at the waist or hips.
2. Knee flexion should not exceed 90 degrees when weight-bearing.
3. Watch the platform periodically.
4. Focus on the feet first. Add arm movements when proficient with the footwork.
5. Step to the center of the step. Don't let your feet hang off the edge.
6. Stay close to the platform as you step down.
7. Don't step down with you back to the platform.
8. Step lightly. Avoid pounding your feet on the step.
9. Allow your whole foot to contact the floor and step (except during propulsion movements).
10. Use proper lifting techniques and carrry the step close to the body.

III. Guidelines for Various Levels

A. Stage 1

Someone who has not participated in a reular exercise program.

Step Height: 4 inches*
Stepping Duration: 10 minutes

B. Stage 2

A regular exerciser who is new to step training.

Step Height: up to 6 inches*
Stepping Duration: 10 minutes

C. Stage 3

A regular stepper.

Step Height: up to 8 inches*
Stepping Duration: 20 minutes

D. Stage 4

A highly skilled and regular stepper.

Step Height: up to 10 inches*
Stepping Duration: 20+ minutes

When selecting a step height, be sure the weight-bearing knee does not flex beyond 90 degrees.

IV. Class Format

A. Pre-Class Instruction

Duration: 2-3 minutes
Purpose: To familiarize participants with step training technique and guidelines.

B. Warm-Up

Tempo: 120-134 bpm
Duration: 8-12 minutes
Purpose: To prepare the body for exercise.

C. Aerobics

Tempo: 118-122 bpm*
Duration: 20-30 minutes
Purpose: To improve cardiovascular fitness, decrease body fat; caloric expenditure.

*126 bpm may be appropriate for highly skilled steppers as long as proper alignment and technique is maintained.

D. Isolation

Tempo 120-130 bpm
Duration: 5-30 minutes
Purpose: To improve muscular strength and endurance.

D. Cool-Down/Flexibility

Tempo: up to 100 bpm
Duration: 5-10 minutes
Purpose: To improve flexibility and make sure participants have adequately cooled down before leaving class.